Alexander Kennedy

Amazon.com/author/alexanderkennedy

*Copyright © 2017 Fritzen Publishing LLC.
All Rights Reserved.*

Alexander Kennedy is an imprint owned by Fritzen Publishing LLC.

No part of this book may be reproduced or transmitted in any form or by any means, electronic or mechanical, including photocopying, recording or by any information storage and retrieval system, without written permission from the publisher.

The information provided within this book is for general informational purposes only. While we try to keep the information up-to-date and correct, there are no representations or warranties, express or implied, about the completeness, accuracy, reliability, suitability or availability with respect to the information, products, services, or related graphics contained in this book for any purpose.

Have a question or concern? Let us know.
FritzenPublishing.com | support@fritzenpublishing.com

Contents

Prologue 5
Chapter 1: The Boy from Hyde Park 15
Chapter 2: Political Beginnings 31
Chapter 3: From the Ashes 49
Chapter 4: Roosevelt in '32 67
Chapter 5: Fighting for the Nation 93
Chapter 6: Fighting for the World 155
Epilogue 203
Sources 207

Prologue

The two men barely spoke as the car made its way to the Capitol. One was Herbert Hoover, the sitting President of the United States, the "Great Engineer" elected to succeed Calvin Coolidge and oversee the economy's seemingly endless march upward. The second was Franklin D. Roosevelt, an aristocratic New York politician who had left office as governor two months before.

On paper, it should have been Hoover, not Roosevelt, who would become one of the great presidents of U.S. history. Hoover entered office with qualifications that few politicians of his generation could match. The son of a Quaker store-owner, Hoover left his native Iowa for Stanford University, where he received a geology degree. He then traveled the world as a mining engineer and witnessed China's proto-nationalist Boxer Rebellion, during which he aided U.S. Marines in rescuing stranded Americans. His textbook

Principles of Mining became the standard in its field, and his mining consultancy proved so profitable that he retired in 1914 as a multimillionaire, having just turned 40.

Always seeking to be of service, Hoover then turned his attention to charity. He helped Americans escape the outbreak of World War I in Europe, and when Belgium experienced a food crisis following German occupation, he organized a massively successful relief effort. Thanks to Hoover's publicity, "starving Belgians" soon became a dinner-table threat to reluctant children in the same way "starving Africans" would be for a later generation. His work made him internationally famous and revered; the famous Russian writer Maxim Gorky wrote Hoover that "You have saved from death 3,5000,000 children and 5,500,000 adults." Even a young Franklin Roosevelt wrote privately of his desire that Hoover (whose party preferences were not yet known) would someday become President of the United States: "There could not be a better one."

Though both parties pursued Hoover as a candidate, he was appointed Secretary of Commerce by Republican President Warren G. Harding. Hoover continued in this post for eight years, through Harding's sudden death and the subsequent Coolidge administration. The Great Mississippi Flood of 1927, the worst in U.S. history, gave Hoover another opportunity to show his genius for disaster relief, and when Coolidge announced his intention not to run for re-election in 1928, Hoover's succession to the office was all but guaranteed. The Democrats deepened their troubles by nominating New York Governor Al Smith, who was Catholic and therefore rejected by the party's Southern wing. Hoover promised voters "a chicken in every pot and a car in every garage" and swept into office in a landslide.

But the Great Engineer soon found the machinery of the economy running out of control. Stock prices began to fall in his first year in office, culminating in the "Black Tuesday" crash of October 29, 1929. The volatility soon spread worldwide. In 1930 a slight upturn caused Hoover to unwisely declare "we have passed the worst," but unemployment continued to grow while the GDP shrank. The midterm elections turned out the Republican majorities of each houses, and Hoover soon found himself facing a Democratic-led Congress determined to oppose any relief measures he proposed. Even members of his own party began to defect, and Hoover's famously aloof personality prevented him from rallying either Washington or the country around a coherent plan. In the words of historian David M.

Kennedy, "1931 thus marked a long season of solitary presidential combat against the massing forces of the nation's greatest economic disaster."

A series of banking failures in 1930, '31, and '32 continued to devastate the economy, and in July 1932, thousands of desperate World War I veterans seeking early payment of their service bonuses marched on Washington. When police asked for federal help to clear the protestors' camp, Hoover authorized General Douglas MacArthur to contain the situation. Against his subordinate Dwight D. Eisenhower's advice, MacArthur exceeded his orders by commanding Major George Patton's cavalry to charge the veterans with tear gas and tanks. The resulting violence, in which the infant child of a "Bonus Army" marcher was killed, cemented Hoover's reputation for heartlessness. By now, the shantytowns of the homeless were called "Hoovervilles," and the newspapers these unfortunates slept beneath were called "Hoover blankets." Despite all his seeming gifts, Hoover's presidency was doomed. Polls of modern historians rank him only just above disastrous presidencies like those of James Buchanan, Richard Nixon, and Andrew Johnson.

But to Hoover's left in the car that day was a man who future historians, and future generations, would consider one of America's two or three greatest leaders. Little before now had suggested that Roosevelt would someday be considered a giant of U.S. history. Where Hoover had been a self-made man, Roosevelt was a patrician with an elite education; where Hoover was an internationally known businessman and humanitarian, Roosevelt was a professional politician; where Hoover had literally written the book about his field, Roosevelt hardly ever read a book at all, preferring to gather ideas from conversation.

Supreme Court Justice Oliver Wendell Holmes famously described Roosevelt as having a "second-class intellect, but a first-class temperament." Yet where Hoover had failed, Roosevelt would--after great difficulty--succeed. His second-class intellect and first-class temperament would lead the nation for a little more than twelve years, seeing it out of the Great Depression and through the greatest armed conflict of its history.

All this lay in the future, however. Today the nation still lay in crisis, its banking system at a total standstill. The governor of Illinois and Roosevelt's replacement as governor of New York were so pressed by emergency financial business that they could not even attend the inauguration. General MacArthur, still in charge of Washington security, had deployed machine guns along the inaugural parade route in anticipation of a riot.

The parade reached the Capitol, where a crowd of a hundred thousand waited to hear the man in whom the United States had now invested so many hopes. Despite the cold, Roosevelt ascended to the East Portico without coat or hat. When the clock struck noon, Chief Justice Charles Evans Hughes, later to be Roosevelt's great enemy, led the new president in the oath of office. Roosevelt stepped to the podium and began his inaugural address with the famous words: "Let me assert my firm belief that the only thing we have to fear is fear itself."

The day was March 4, 1933, and Roosevelt had just stepped firmly into history.

Chapter 1: The Boy from Hyde Park

Child of Privilege

Franklin D. Roosevelt was a child of privilege. The Roosevelts had been in New York state since before there was a New York state, and one ancestor had even served in the American Revolution. His mother's family, the Delanos, also had a name of long standing: Columbus Delano had been an election manager for Abraham Lincoln and a cabinet secretary for Ulysses S. Grant, and Herman Melville based his great novella "Benito Cereno" on the memoirs of Captain Amasa Delano. Franklin's maternal grandfather, Warren Delano, had made a killing in the shady Chinese opium trade, while Franklin's paternal grandfather had grown wealthy from real estate investments.

Franklin's father James--nicknamed "Squire James" for his constant formality--invested wisely in railroads and coal, and moved at the highest levels of New York society. After the death of his first wife Rebecca in 1876, James married his sixth cousin, Sara Ann Delano. Their only child, Franklin D. Roosevelt, was born two years after the wedding, on January 30, 1882. (James had a much older son from his previous marriage, also named James, but the younger James had already married and moved out when Franklin was born.)

Sara, who had been a spoiled child herself, doted on Franklin to an extraordinary degree. His early life consisted of cosseting and luxury, with his parents splitting their time between Europe and their New York estate at Hyde Park. In their travels, Franklin picked up basic German and French, skills that would serve him well in the war years of his presidency. Because James was already a sick man, suffering a serious heart condition that periodically left him an invalid, the family often traveled to spas like Bad Nauheim.

Franklin also learned to move in elite circles, picking up the distinctive but hard-to-define accent of his later life: vaguely New England, vaguely British, and vaguely rich. Legend holds that at the age of 5, his father once took him to meet Democratic U.S. President Grover Cleveland. Cleveland, who was then battling a Republican-controlled Senate over tariffs, told the boy, "My little man, I am making a strange wish for you. It is that you may never be president of the United States." Franklin's greatest loves as a boy were stamp collecting and sailing, hobbies he would pursue throughout his life. He was thrilled when his family built a cottage and began regularly to summer at Campobello Island, where they kept a cutter called the Half Moon.

As historian H.W. Brands observes, one aspect of Franklin's childhood would have severe consequences for his adult life: his isolation from other children. Though Franklin received endless attention from his doting mother and the family servants--he was never lonely--he grew up without siblings and largely without playmates. As a result, he was never exposed to most childhood illnesses, with long-term consequences for the development of his immune system. Though polio's etiology has never been fully understood, doctors noted during many outbreaks that children of wealthy neighborhoods seemed more vulnerable than those of less sanitary poor neighborhoods. By missing out on these early illnesses, Franklin was probably made more vulnerable to the disease that would one day rob him of his legs.

Groton and Harvard

At 14, Franklin was sent to Groton School, a Massachusetts boarding school run by the Episcopalian priest Endicott Peabody. Groton was an elite school for elite children, financially supported by banker J.P. Morgan and with allies like rising New York political star Theodore Roosevelt (Franklin's fifth cousin). Peabody set his charges to a character-building regime of early mornings, hard work, and cold-water bathing. Most importantly, he sought to instill a sense of public service in his charges, arguing that the sons of privilege must help the less fortunate.

Peabody's message resonated intensely with Roosevelt, though biographers continue to debate whether his Groton experience reshaped his character or simply revealed traits that were already there. Roosevelt himself said of Peabody that "as long as I live, his influence will mean more to me than that of any other people next to my father and mother." Later Groton graduates would include Harry Truman's secretary of state Dean Acheson, and New York governor and diplomat W. Averell Harriman. For his role in teaching so many members of the future Establishment, Peabody would later be described by TIME as "the most famous headmaster of his generation." When Roosevelt later chose schools for his own sons, all four went to Groton.

Franklin's elderly, invalid father died in 1900, with his two sons by his side. The same year, Franklin graduated from Groton and enrolled in Harvard, majoring in history. (His mother Sara, now solely devoted to her son's well-being, moved to Boston to stay near him.) Roosevelt was an unexceptional student academically, but extraordinary socially. Discovering his gifts for leadership, he became the editor of the Harvard Crimson and was accepted to several elite clubs. In 1904, he won his first election victory to become chairman of his class.

In this same period, following the assassination of William McKinley, Franklin's cousin Theodore assumed the presidency of the United States. In 1904, he won re-election in his own right, the first vice president to do so since Martin Van Buren in 1837. The young Franklin watched his cousin's success from afar, silently planning for his own life to follow the same track.

Eleanor

Franklin and Eleanor were never sure when they had first met. Eleanor was Franklin's sixth cousin, the daughter of Theodore Roosevelt's brother Elliott. (Bearing the name Roosevelt from birth, she would be the only First Lady in U.S. history to have the same name after her wedding as before.) They were told by relatives that they had played together as children--she was two years younger than he--but neither could remember this themselves.

As they grew older, they sometimes danced together at Christmas parties given by relatives.

These were moments that Eleanor did remember, and treasure, because her own childhood was a misery. Her father and several uncles were alcoholics, and Eleanor had to lock her bedroom door at night to protect herself from them. In addition to her brothers Elliot, Jr., and Hall, Eleanor had a half-brother who had been conceived when her father impregnated a servant girl, creating a public scandal. Eleanor's mother Anna was a society beauty who treated her homely daughter harshly. The family's dysfunction left Eleanor so unhappy and serious that her mother nicknamed her "Granny."

Things only got worse. Anna died of diphtheria when Eleanor was eight years old, and her younger brother Elliot, Jr. died of the same disease not long after. Her father Elliott, who was in and out of sanitariums to treat his alcoholism, finally died in 1894, when Eleanor was nine. During a fit of delirium tremens, he had injured himself trying to leap from a window and then died of a seizure. Eleanor was sent to live with her maternal grandmother, who had no affection for the girl. The only survivor of her immediate family, Eleanor's youngest brother Hall, would later succumb to the same alcoholism that killed their father, dying while Eleanor was First Lady.

From 1899 to 1902, Eleanor boarded at a British finishing school, run by the well-known feminist educator Marie Souvestre, the daughter of French philosopher Emile Souvestre. From Mme. Souvestre, Eleanor learned independent thinking, self-respect, and ideals of public service. She also came out of her shell socially, finding herself--to her surprise--quite popular among her classmates. When her grandmother ordered her back to America to "come out" as a debutante instead of finishing her studies, Eleanor returned, but only grudgingly. This return put her back in her future husband's path.

Courtship and Marriage

In the summer of 1902, Franklin spotted Eleanor on a commuter train, and the two passed the journey together. They briefly lost touch but saw each other again at a family party in early 1903, and soon a secret courtship began. Franklin had had a similar romance the previous year, with another society girl named Alice Sohier; he even proposed marriage, though he never discussed her with his mother. When her parents discovered the clandestine correspondence, however, they whisked her away to Europe, figuring rightly that Franklin would lose interest. Eleanor was not going anywhere, however. One day during their courtship, Franklin visited an immigrant aid group at which Eleanor was a volunteer teacher. It was perhaps his first exposure to serious poverty and marked the beginning of a new social awareness in him. On a joint visit to Groton, where Eleanor's brother Hall was now enrolled, Franklin proposed marriage.

One formidable obstacle still remained, however: Franklin's intensely possessive mother. When told during the 1903 Thanksgiving holiday of the engagement, Sara opposed it immediately. Now it was Sara's turn to send her child on vacation, taking him on a long Caribbean holiday in a desperate ploy to delay the couple's engagement announcement. But Eleanor was more steadfast than her fiancé had been in similar circumstances, and Franklin was no less determined to marry her on his return.

Why was Eleanor so appealing to the flirtatious, handsome Franklin despite her "ugly duckling" reputation? In cold political terms, marrying the niece of a sitting president advances any young politician's prospects--never mind that the president in question was Franklin's personal hero. But despite the collapse of their marriage a decade later, most biographers judge the marriage to have been a love match at first. Franklin admired Eleanor's intellect and social conscience, and seems to have seen in her, even at this early date, the world-changing woman she could become. Nor was Eleanor as unattractive to men as she self-disparagingly claimed. When she agreed to marry Franklin, she had at least three other serious suitors, one of whom was so devastated that he could barely write her the socially-mandated congratulations on her engagement.

Eleanor also seems to have glimpsed Franklin's potential, despite his mediocre scholarship and lack of career plans. She was aware of his reputation for drinking and womanizing, but even these may not have hurt his chances with her; Eleanor saw something of her dead father in Franklin and desired to protect him. According to biographer Blanche Wiesen Cook, Eleanor was at this time infatuated with George Bernard Shaw's play Candida, the story of a woman who gives her love to the man who needs her the most, but only if he acknowledges her as an equal party. This plot foreshadowed much of her marriage to Franklin, particularly her role in rebuilding his political career after his polio infection.

In late 1904--a year after first becoming engaged--Franklin at last persuaded his mother to allow him to announce the engagement. The wedding was eventually fixed for St. Patrick's Day, 1905, to allow the president to attend and give away the bride while also courting New York's Irish vote. Franklin's former headmaster, Endicott Peabody, presided. The wedding ceremony was not a success; Theodore's Secret Service protection threw the preparations into chaos, and Theodore drew the attention of both press and guests away from the couple to himself. Franklin and Eleanor soon found themselves standing alone at their own wedding party.

During the same period, Franklin graduated from Harvard and went on to Columbia Law School. It was what his cousin Theodore had done, after all.

Chapter 2:
Political Beginnings

A Four-Point Plan

Though he realized the value of a law degree for his political prospects, Roosevelt had little enthusiasm for his studies. Biographer Jean Edward Smith records one of Roosevelt's professors as stating that he "had little aptitude for the law and 'made no effort to overcome that handicap by hard work.'" His Columbia transcripts reveal many absences and mediocre overall marks, including two courses that he failed and had to retake.

In the summer of 1905, Franklin and Eleanor took a three-month honeymoon in Europe, during which Eleanor became pregnant for the first time. By letter, they urged Franklin's mother Sara to arrange a home for them on their return. As it turned out, Sara bought not one home, but two: she commissioned adjoining townhouses, one for the newlyweds and one for herself. Eleanor had allowed her husband and mother-in-law to make these arrangements, but she broke down in tears not long after moving in, resenting Sara's control of their lives.

The mutual dislike between the two most important women of Roosevelt's life (or two of three, if one counts Lucy Mercer) deepened into a quiet, lifelong feud. In an unpublished bit of memoir, Eleanor later wrote:

She [Sara] determined to bend the marriage to the way she wanted it to be. What she wanted was to hold on to Franklin and his children; she wanted them to grow as she wished. As it turned out, Franklin's children were more my mother-in-law's children than they were mine.

The couple's oldest son James remembered his grandmother once telling him the same, in almost identical words: "Your mother only bore you, I am more your mother than your mother is."

In fact, despite the couple's six children (one of whom died in infancy), Eleanor had little enthusiasm for motherhood and even less aptitude for it. On one occasion, zealously following a parenting trend for giving babies "fresh air," she left Anna (the couple's oldest daughter) crying in a box in the cold outdoors until the Roosevelts' neighbors threatened to inform the Society for the Prevention of Cruelty to Children. Franklin, in turn, was a detached father who would occasionally romp with his children but left all discipline to Eleanor and Sara.

In 1907, Franklin passed the New York State Bar exam, but he dropped out of Columbia afterward without completing his degree. In September of that year, he apprenticed himself to Carter, Ledyard, and Milburn, a well-respected practice on Wall Street that represented Standard Oil, J. P. Morgan, and other giants. FDR had little interest in the work and was frank with his fellow apprentices about his desire to go into politics instead.

At this time, Roosevelt famously confided in a friend his four-point plan to become President of the United States. First he would be elected to the New York State Assembly; then he would be appointed Secretary of the Navy; then he would be elected Governor of New York; using the governorship to draw national attention, he would then make a run at the presidency. It's no coincidence that this was exactly the same route his cousin Theodore's career had taken, excepting TR's interlude in the Spanish-American War. As it turned out, Franklin also would trace this precise path to the summit of power.

State Senator

His first chance came in 1910. The political parties of this era were much less unified in their ideology than the parties of today, and both Republicans and Democrats had progressive and conservative wings. In the Republican party, these two wings were about to go to war, with ex-president Teddy Roosevelt leading the progressives in a revolt against his supposedly more conservative successor and former close friend, President William Howard Taft. With the Republican party self-destructing and the progressives in ascendance among Democrats, the time was ripe for a progressive Democrat like Franklin to strike. He put his name in for a state senate seat that had been held by the Republicans in every term since the Civil War, but he nonetheless won handily. Democrats swept the state and the nation, taking control of governorships, state legislatures, and the U.S. Congress.

Roosevelt had put himself on the front of an important wave, and he worked quickly to consolidate his reputation as a young man to watch. Unlike many state legislators, he moved his family to Albany. At this time, state legislatures elected U.S. Senators (this would be changed only three years later by the Seventeenth Amendment), and the first order of business for the new Democratic majority was to replace an outgoing Republican.

This meant, in practical terms, that the new senator for New York state would be appointed by the boss of Tammany Hall. New York's Democratic Party had been dominated by the corrupt Tammany Hall organization for a century, as far back as the days of Aaron Burr. The current boss, Charles Murphy, proposed a Tammany Hall crony and former lieutenant governor for the open senate seat. But the progressives saw a chance to flex their newfound muscle in the party, proposing a reform candidate instead. (Roosevelt soon found himself the de facto leader of this "insurgency" (as the newspapers of the day called it)) for two reasons: his famous name, which put him atop every news story, and his large Albany house, which gave the progressives a headquarters at which to meet and plot.

Murphy and Roosevelt clashed in the press throughout the winter, and eventually settled on a compromise candidate that saved face for both men. But even if the battle was a tactical draw, it resulted in a massive strategic victory for Roosevelt. He had emerged as the leader of progressive New York Democrats; he had received months of national press attention; he had taken on the boss of Tammany Hall and emerged unscathed. Perhaps most importantly, he had permanently disassociated himself from New York corruption in the public mind and established a reputation as a courageous reformer.

Assistant Secretary of the Navy

This reputation paid swift dividends. Roosevelt was re-elected in 1912 with the help of his new political consultant, a brilliant, repulsive, chain-smoking little gnome of a man named Louis Howe. Howe's face had been badly scarred in a childhood accident, and Roosevelt did not let them appear in public together, but behind the scenes Howe-- previously a savvy political reporter--would be the mastermind of every Roosevelt election for the next twenty years.

Meanwhile, the Republican civil war culminated in the 1912 presidential election, in which Theodore Roosevelt broke with Taft to form the independent "Bull Moose Party." With the Republican vote badly split, the Democrats captured the White House with a relative political novice, former president of Princeton University and Governor of New Jersey Woodrow Wilson. As a rising progressive star, Franklin had headed Wilson's New York committee, and he was soon approached by new Secretary of the Navy Josephus Daniels and offered the post of Assistant Secretary--the second step of Franklin's own master plans. Most Democratic politicians were so weak on naval affairs, it turned out, that Franklin's childhood sailing experience alone had made him more qualified for the post than any of his rivals.

As Assistant Secretary of the Navy, Roosevelt carefully cultivated Navy officials as well as the labor unions that worked in the shipyards. He later stated that the most important accomplishment of his term was that "we did not have one single major dispute--no strike, no walk-out, or serious trouble in all of the navy yards all over the United States." In 1914, World War I began in Europe, and Wilson began to build up the navy in anticipation of trouble. Roosevelt oversaw much of this expansion, as well as the explosion of new ship-building when the U.S. formally entered the war in 1917 following the sinking of the Lusitania and the discovery of the "Zimmermann Telegram." From this experience, he learned valuable lessons in wartime procurement and organization, lessons he would later put to use in fighting his own world war.

The End of the Affair

In 1918, Roosevelt went on a tour of Europe to inspect American naval facilities. On the return voyage, he caught the H1N1 flu virus (the so-called "Spanish flu"), which had reached epidemic proportions thanks to the disruptions and dislocations of war. Five hundred million people around the world were made sick, and as many as one hundred million died, perhaps five percent of the global population at the time. Roosevelt would survive, but his illness still had a surprising cost. As Eleanor unpacked her delirious husband's luggage, she made a discovery that effectively ended their marriage: a packet of love letters to Franklin from Eleanor's social secretary, Lucy Mercer.

Mercer had been born in 1891 to upper-class parents who then lost everything in the Panic of 1893. She worked as a dress shop as a young woman before Eleanor hired her as a secretary. Her affair with Franklin had probably been going on for more than two years before Eleanor's discovery, and some of the Roosevelts' circle were already aware of it. Theodore's daughter Alice even made a point to invite Franklin and Mercer to luncheons together, telling friends that "he deserved a good time... he was married to Eleanor." (Alice's cruelty to her younger cousin was legendary in Washington society).

What happened immediately after Eleanor's discovery is not well understood, but the Roosevelts' children later said that Eleanor offered Franklin an uncontested divorce. Surprisingly, Franklin seriously considered taking it, though in the moral climate of his day, it would have permanently destroyed his political ambitions. Of all people, it seems to have been Sara who "saved" the Roosevelts' marriage. Despite her resentment of Eleanor, the potential scandal of Franklin's abandoning his wife to marry Mercer was far worse. Sara threatened to cut Franklin off financially for good if he went through with his plan. Louis Howe also pleaded with Franklin not to squander their success in building his national image. Between his mother and Howe, Franklin finally backed down.

From this day forward, Franklin and Eleanor's relationship becomes hard for biographers to define. Eleanor insisted that Franklin end the affair with Mercer, and he did so, at least for a time. Franklin and Eleanor slept in separate bedrooms for the rest of their lives, and they never had another child. James Roosevelt described his parents' later marriage as "an armed truce that endured until the day he died." Yet in other ways the two remained emotionally close, or even closer. Franklin made more of a point to spend time with

Eleanor and the children, and she made more of an effort to participate in his social life.

The incident led Eleanor to fundamentally rethink her role in Franklin's life. Unhappy as a mother and a wife, she needed to recreate herself as something new. Louis Howe began to tutor her in politics, and she took a more active interest in world affairs, setting the stage for her precedent-breaking activism as First Lady. From the disaster of the Lucy Mercer affair was born the Eleanor Roosevelt the world would later come to revere.

The Newport Sex Scandal and the Democratic Ticket

Not long after his marriage nearly collapsed, a scandal threatened Franklin Roosevelt's political career. As part of the progressives' fight against prostitution, Roosevelt had ordered the creation of an undercover investigative unit at the Newport, Rhode Island, naval training facility. Unbeknownst to Roosevelt, the unit soon expanded its investigation to homosexuality as well, and its members were ordered to participate in homosexual acts with base personnel to get enough evidence for convictions. (Because even the scandal's investigators could not speak explicitly and factually about homosexuality at the time, the extent of these "acts" remains a matter of conjecture.) When an Episcopalian priest was caught in the sting, the scandal exploded into the national press. Roosevelt was criticized for his role in the investigation and did little to help himself by going on the attack with several libel suits.

But the bad press proved only temporary. When the 1920 Democratic National Convention met to pick Woodrow Wilson's potential successor, they settled on Ohio governor James M. Cox on the 44th ballot. Because Cox leaned to the conservative wing of the party, a nationally known progressive was a logical choice to balance the ticket. Roosevelt soon learned he had been named the Democratic vice presidential candidate.

In his acceptance speech, Roosevelt heartily endorsed Wilsonian ideals, particularly the creation of League of Nations, an international organization proposed by Wilson to peacefully resolve disputes that might otherwise lead to war. But the League was deeply unpopular among the American people and had been blocked in the Senate by the Republican Henry Cabot Lodge. Though Roosevelt surely had few illusions about his party's chances, he campaigned like a demon, making nearly a thousand speeches in support of Cox, Wilson's legacy, and the Democratic Party.

The speeches made no discernible difference. Cox and Roosevelt were soundly defeated by Ohio Senator Warren G. Harding and strikebreaking Massachusetts Governor Calvin Coolidge. In the worst defeat of the party's history, the Democratic ticket carried only 11 of 48 states and lost by a popular vote of 16 million to 9 million. Cox's reputation never recovered, and he never held office again. But despite the loss, and despite the still-simmering Newport Sex Scandal, Roosevelt was still regarded by many as a future star.

At least, that is, until he contracted polio.

Chapter 3:
From the Ashes

After the Defeat

After his failed run at the vice presidency, Roosevelt became a Wall Street lawyer once more. He worked for several years for the New York office of the Fidelity and Deposit Company of Maryland; he would leave in 1924 to form a partnership with a younger lawyer named Basil O'Connor. (Basil O'Connor was born Daniel O'Connor, but started going by his more distinctive middle name after seeing the endless list of Daniel O'Connors in the New York phone directory.) O'Connor did most of the firm's work, and in later life, would become nationally famous for founding the March of Dimes and funding Jonas Salk's research into a polio vaccine.

Franklin threw himself back into New York society, joining the boards of a wide range of charitable and civic organizations. Under Louis Howe's patient tutelage, Eleanor took her first political steps as well. Most notably, she joined several organizations of women voters, a constituency she would cultivate for her husband throughout their lives together. Meanwhile, Franklin periodically traveled to Washington to face Congressional subcommittees in the ongoing Newport Sex Scandal investigation.

No serious evidence of wrongdoing by Roosevelt was ever found, but in any case, the scandal was soon the least of his problems. On the family's next vacation, he found himself fighting for his life.

Onset

It remains unclear exactly how Franklin D. Roosevelt was infected with polio. In fact, a small minority of medical historians have argued that Roosevelt fell ill not with polio, but with Guillain-Barré Syndrome, an autoimmune disorder that sometimes follows bacterial infection. However, the majority of biographers agree with the polio diagnosis of Roosevelt's doctors, and this book will follow their lead in referring to his paralytic disease as "polio."

Assuming it was polio, then--a disease that primarily affects children--how did the thirty-nine-year-old Roosevelt catch it? As noted above, Roosevelt's isolated childhood meant that he probably lacked immunity to many childhood diseases. A child with many other children around had a much better chance of being exposed to weakened or dead polio virus--the same strategy later used to vaccinate against the disease--from the stool of infected children.

For reasons still not understood, the disease seemed to flourish in hot summers like that of 1921. A Boy Scout camp near the Roosevelts' vacation home, Campobello, may have provided the vector for infection, as an infected child played in the water of the Hudson River. Many more children picnicked in the nearby Bear Mountain State Park, a gift of the Harriman family to New York State. As historian James Tobin catalogues, the possibility for infection was almost endless: Roosevelt may have shaken a sick boy's hand, or shared a piece of food touched by an infected child, or drank contaminated water.

Though no outbreak of polio was reported among the children at Bear Mountain that week, Roosevelt may have been unusually vulnerable. Not only did he probably lack ordinary immunity, but he also was exhausted and angry from another round of Congressional hearings on Newport. But however Roosevelt ingested the virus, it soon flamed through his body.

The first symptom was a chill, and Franklin went to bed early that night, believing he had a simple cold. The next day he awoke feverish and with a partially paralyzed left leg. A local doctor examined him and agreed with Franklin that he was only having an extreme reaction to a cold, but as the day progressed, Franklin began to lose the use of his arms and legs. The polio virus was now replicating in, and forever destroying, his motor neurons.

With Eleanor increasingly concerned, Louis Howe (also along for the Roosevelt family holiday) found a vacationing surgeon to examine Franklin in secret to give a second opinion. Though no one gave it much thought at the time, this was the first step in what would be a lifelong campaign to conceal the extent of Franklin's paralysis from the American public. The surgeon suspected polio, and ordered Howe and Eleanor to begin a course of painful massages of Franklin's legs to try to preserve blood flow to the muscles. New England's leading polio expert was brought and confirmed the diagnosis.

At this point, Roosevelt was recovering. It was clear he would survive, and the doctors even gave him hope that he might walk again someday. Roosevelt held onto this hope for the next twenty-five years, never accepting that his paralysis might be permanent. But it was.

Recuperation

Howe never lost faith in the prospects of a Roosevelt comeback, and he carefully managed the press in the months following Franklin's illness. He informed the New York Times that Roosevelt had been sick, but was "improving." In a later story, also managed by Howe, doctors explicitly and falsely assured the public that Roosevelt was "not crippled."

Roosevelt himself remained in seclusion until he could keep up his end of the ruse. During these years of recovery, Eleanor and Howe became Franklin's eyes, ears, and public face. Eleanor represented her husband at social events, while Howe continued to handle the backroom negotiating that kept Franklin's political career alive.

Franklin and Howe agreed that the public needed to be at least partly deceived about his paralysis for him to have any chance at the presidency. With agonizing effort, Roosevelt therefore trained himself to fake a sort of walking by strapping iron braces to his legs and, while using a cane for support, swiveling his torso back and forth to lurch his legs forward. Howe and Roosevelt's later staff went to extraordinary lengths to avoid having Roosevelt appear in public in his wheelchair, and the national press proved surprisingly cooperative. Despite the tens of thousands of photographs taken of Roosevelt in his lifetime, the number of photographs showing his wheelchair can literally be counted on one hand.

With Roosevelt semi-ambulatory, it was time to present him to the public again. In 1924, he chaired the presidential campaign of Al Smith of New York, the Catholic nominee who in four years would win the Democratic nomination only to be soundly defeated by Hoover. Smith would not be the candidate this year, however. The 1924 Democratic convention deadlocked in unprecedented fashion between Smith and William McAdoo, Woodrow Wilson's son-in-law, Secretary of the Treasury, and spiritual successor. After a bitter fourteen days and 103 ballots, the convention at last compromised on John W. Davis, a conservative Wall Street lawyer. The Democratic ticket that year won only 21% of the popular vote, barely ahead of a third-party challenge by progressive Republican Robert "Fightin' Bob" La Follette of Wisconsin.

But, as in 1920, what was a disaster for the party was a personal triumph for Roosevelt. He stood on the convention floor in his iron braces for every one of those fourteen days, proving his health in the most public way possible. He also delivered the nominating speech for Smith before the convention. Roosevelt gambled heavily on his long, painful walk to the podium that day. One slip or stumble, one public show of his weakness, and his political prospects could have died on the spot. But Roosevelt reached the podium smiling and radiating good health, and his speech was a triumph, a widely acknowledged highlight of a failed convention.

The appearance catapulted Roosevelt back onto the national stage. Once vulnerable to (somewhat accurate) charges of being a spoiled aristocrat, Roosevelt now possessed a genuinely heroic narrative of disaster and recovery. Smith's rise to national prominence meant that he might soon be leaving the New York governorship, leaving the path clear for Roosevelt to claim it for himself. And many Democrats began to see this talented, still young politician as the man who could unite a badly fractured party. Summing up the events, the New York Times called him "the most popular man in the convention."

Years of Waiting

Following the 1924 election, Roosevelt sought to put his new prestige to use in healing his party's divisions. The party's Southern wing was deeply conservative and rural, though loyal to the party popularly associated with the Confederacy. In the north, Democrats tended to be progressive and urban, drawing heavily on immigrant areas of the cities (Tammany

Hall is the archetypal example). In the six decades since the Civil War, this fractious coalition had only managed to elect two Democrats to the White House: Grover Cleveland and Woodrow Wilson.

Roosevelt first reached out to populist icon William Jennings Bryan--a three-time loser as Democratic nominee, and the elder statesman of the party's conservative wing. But in 1925, Bryan faced off against Clarence Darrow in the notorious "Scopes monkey trial" over the teaching of evolution, pitting conservatives and progressives against each other once more. Bryan died only weeks after, ending any chance of him and Roosevelt coming together.

Meanwhile, Roosevelt continued his recuperation. In 1921, he had hired a personal secretary named Marguerite "Missy" LeHand, who would remain indispensable to him until she suffered a stroke twenty years later.

Between 1924 and 1927, he spent his winters in Florida, on a houseboat called the Larocco. LeHand served as his hostess, Eleanor having tried living on the boat for only a week before giving up. LeHand and Franklin became very close, and their contemporaries--like later biographers--often debated whether the pair were romantically and sexually involved. (Biographers also continue to debate whether Franklin's partial paralysis left him capable of sexual activity, and the question has never been conclusively resolved.) When Roosevelt sold this boat after 1927, putting an end to their travels together, LeHand had a nervous breakdown so extreme that she required hospitalization.

During this period, Roosevelt discovered the spa of Warm Springs, Georgia--the waters of which were rumored to cure polio--and he and LeHand would travel here each spring at the end of their boat trip. Though the waters never cured him, Roosevelt made this town his home away from Hyde Park and would one day die there. In 1926, he purchased a Warm Springs resort and founded a hydrotherapy center for polio victims; it still operates today as the Roosevelt Warm Springs Institute for Rehabilitation. Eleanor hated the resort as much as she had the Larocco, and rarely accompanied her husband there.

Another Governor Roosevelt

Seeing no other legitimate option, Roosevelt again backed Al Smith in 1928. Though Smith's Catholicism and "wet" (anti-temperance) stance were anathema to the party's Southern wing, Roosevelt believed he was still the party's best shot at the presidency. But Smith was also New York's governor at the time, which left Roosevelt with a conundrum.

1928 was shaping up to be a terrible year for Democrats. The Republican boom was still in full swing and the party was split over Smith; the effects were expected to be felt in every race of the coming cycle. Both Howe and Eleanor advised him against running for governor in this hostile season. Nor was Rooscvelt's re-entry to public life quite complete, and his mother had pressured him ever since his illness to retire and live a life like his father's, a local "squire."

But Roosevelt had long coveted the governorship of New York as the final step in his road to the presidency, and if he failed to strike now, another man might slip in first. Under extreme pressure from party leaders-- who believed Roosevelt their only chance to keep the office--Franklin defied all those close to him and agreed to run. Republicans immediately attacked his candidacy on health grounds, but Roosevelt put these doubts to rest with a strenuous speaking tour across the state, sometimes giving as many as 14 speeches in a single day. He drew crowds that were far larger than expected, and by election day he was a narrow favorite to win.

On November 6, 1932, the election followed a now-familiar pattern. The situation for the national party was a disaster. Herbert Hoover not only won heavily in the north, but even carried five states of the so-called "Solid South" (named for its traditional loyalty to Democrats). It was the first time these states had opted for a Republican since Reconstruction. Like James Cox and John W. Davis before him, Al Smith's political career was over, wrecked on the fissures of his party. He even lost in his home state of New York.

For a time, Roosevelt's prospects also hung in the balance. His campaign team tracked the tight race throughout the night. He was running ahead of Smith, that was clear, but how far ahead? By 4 AM they finally knew. Roosevelt had won by only 25,000 votes, but he had won. New York had a second Governor Roosevelt, and Franklin had only one step left in his plan: the presidency.

Chapter 4:
Roosevelt in '32

Governor: First Term

Roosevelt had barely been sworn in before he ran into trouble from an unexpected quarter: his long-time ally Al Smith. Having failed to win the White House, Smith had nowhere to move on to, and was not ready to release his hold on Albany just yet. Smith attempted to push his own people--his advisor Belle Moskowitz and future "power broker" Robert Moses--on Roosevelt, believing the younger man would need their guidance. Roosevelt had a famous aversion to face-to-face conflict, and later would be notorious for nodding along and seemingly agreeing with White House guests, only to ignore or contradict their advice the moment after they left the room. He showed this aversion in his discussions with Moskowitz and other Smith people; he never told them to their faces that they wouldn't have jobs, but it became clear no jobs would materialize.

Smith soon realized that Roosevelt had no desire for his help. Amazingly, some biographers have suggested that Smith even failed to realize Roosevelt had designs on the presidency for himself. Though Roosevelt praised his predecessor extravagantly in his inaugural address, Smith soon moved away from Albany, baffled and well on the road to becoming a Roosevelt foe.

As governor, Roosevelt initially focused on farm relief and electricity. Nationally, the agriculture sector was in dire need of help as the Dust Bowl devoured the west. Roosevelt's efforts consequently drew favorable notice well beyond his own state, beginning to endear him to the party's rural wing. He created a gasoline tax that paid for new roads to rural areas, and his rural electrification created cheap energy for impoverished areas. "If the farmer starves today," he said in one speech, "we all starve tomorrow."

Lacking a majority in the state assembly, Roosevelt was forced to adopt a nonpartisan, conciliatory stance in fighting for legislation, further honing his political talents. He also introduced an innovation for which he would later be famous: a regular Sunday night radio broadcast, or "fireside chat". With the increasingly popular technology of radio, Roosevelt found he could bypass his opposition in Albany by appealing to the people directly; his listeners would then pressure their assemblymen, hastening the passage of any Roosevelt-sponsored legislation.

Positioning for the Presidency

Reporters and politicians of the time saw any governor of New York as a potential White House challenger. New York had been known to swing elections since John Adams lost to Thomas Jefferson in 1800, and New Yorkers were overwhelmingly represented among major-party presidential candidates since the Civil War: Horatio Seymour (1868), Horace Greeley (1872), Samuel J. Tilden (1876), Chester A. Arthur (1880--a vice president who assumed the presidency), Grover Cleveland (1884, 1888, 1892), Theodore Roosevelt (1904, 1912), Alton B. Parker (1904), and Charles Evan Hughes (1916). Little wonder, then, that every speech of New York's charismatic new governor was seen as national news.

It was also becoming clear that 1932 would be a good year for Democrats, every bit as good as 1920, '24, and '28 had been bad. The stock market crash of October 29, 1929--forever known as "Black Tuesday"--had hit America hard, and unemployment was beginning to spread.

America had seen stock market crashes and depressions before, but the economy had soon righted itself, and the devastation had never been this widespread. To many observers, it seemed like the end of capitalism, or even of society itself. In Europe, the Depression's horrors gave rise to fascism and encouraged the spread of communism, and the political center found itself swiftly eroding under the attacks of far right and far left. That America experienced no such turmoil is in large part thanks to the political genius of Franklin D. Roosevelt.

Causes of the Great Depression

The causes of the Great Depression are complex, widely debated, and poorly understood. Why did the "bust" of the boom-bust cycle not start swinging back toward "boom" sooner?

It all began with the stock market bubble that built in the American stock market throughout the 1920s. A decade of steady economic growth had finally sent investors into a frenzy. Banks issued loans to private individuals just so that they could play the stock market, even allowing them to buy stocks on margin. Businesses also began to put their profits into gambling on stocks instead of investing tangibly in their own expansion. At the same time, many industries were showing signs of overproduction, and when the economic slowdown began, they found themselves with massive stockpiles of unsold inventory. When the stock market crash came, all of these speculators were wiped out. Businesses realized they had squandered their profits, and banks found themselves with widespread defaults on their loans.

Another important contributor to the bubble was Montagu Norman, the long-serving

Governor of the Bank of England. Norman was obsessed with the gold standard, an economic theory of the day that sought to keep each currency at a precise exchange rate with gold and one another. (This contrasts with the floating-rate currencies of today like the dollar and euro, which are allowed to change value relative to one another.) Though this theory is now generally discredited, its 1920s adherents believed that if the gold standard ever failed, so would international finance. Norman won a famous debate against John Maynard Keynes by persuading Chancellor of the Exchequer Winston Churchill to maintain the gold standard instead of creating a "managed currency." In support of this system, Benjamin Strong of the New York Federal Reserve Bank kept interest rates low even as speculation blazed out of control, all in an effort to prop up the British pound. Hoover, in contrast, had sensed the growing bubble and was furious with the Fed's actions, but he had no tools available with which to deflate it.

Still, as historian David M. Kennedy observes, at least 97% of the population owned no stock, and so the impact of this crash was still limited to a small minority. Unfortunately for the world, that minority was the banks. 1930 saw the first wave of bank failures, and this was where the trouble really began. The National Bank of Kentucky was the first to go, followed by dozens of others. Worst of all was the failure of the so-called Bank of the United States, a private bank with no relationship to the government. This wiped out the savings of 400,000 people at a stroke, and through its name, created the misimpression that the government itself was bankrupt. The actual Federal Reserve was rudderless and uncertain, and failed to inject new money to get commerce moving again.

At the same time, Europe was struggling with problems of its own that dated from World War I. In the 1919 Treaty of Versailles that ended the war, Britain and France had demanded large reparation payments from Germany, 132 billion gold marks. (In this, they followed Germany's own example from the 1870 Franco-Prussian War, in which a proportionately similar sum had been levied against the defeated France. France had paid; Germany never would.) Britain and France, in turn, had incurred massive debts to the U.S. government and U.S. banks.

As the 1920s progressed, war reparations became an increasingly heated issue on both sides of the Atlantic. It was clear to most economists, then as now, that the war debts were hobbling European economies, though the myth that Germany was "crushed" by impossible reparations is generally discounted by historians. Britain and France indicated that they would release Germany from its debts if the U.S. would in turn forgive theirs, but this solution was unpopular with the American people and with many American politicians as well. Calvin Coolidge, on being told of European complaints about the war debt, is reported to have simply replied, "They hired the money, didn't they?" The debt schedule was renegotiated in the 1924 Dawes Plan and the 1928 Young Plan, but the underlying problem remained.

With international finance already choking under the festering debt, the U.S. Congress nonetheless found a way to make things worse. In 1930, it passed the Smoot-Hawley Tariff Act, raising tariffs to record levels; Hoover opposed the measure but eventually signed it into law under pressure from his party. Other nations retaliated with identical tariffs, cutting U.S. imports and exports by as much as 50%.

Under the pressures of war debts, tariffs, the U.S. stock crash and depression, and the maneuvering needed to maintain an artificial gold standard, Europe soon found itself with its own run of bank failures. The Bank of England itself was forced to stop payments, bringing the international economy to a standstill. With no banks to provide loans and savings, and no international markets for manufactured goods, the global economy began a general collapse. By 1932, the world GDP would fall by a staggering 15%.

Hoover's Approach

Though his manner was aloof, Hoover was never the heartless plutocrat of Democratic propaganda, nor was he inactive in the face of the crisis. Hoover initially argued for a volunteer response to the crisis, in which businesses would support the workers in hard times and do their best to stimulate the economy. He also argued that direct aid to individuals would only foster dependence.

But as the crisis wore on, Hoover saw an expanded role for the federal government in managing the economy, going far beyond any of his predecessors in this regard. He proposed countercyclical spending to alleviate the Depression--in today's terms, a "stimulus"--an economic theory only just coming into vogue. He pressured businesses into maintaining wages at 1929 rates, though the agreement only held until 1931. He proposed and passed a federal budget with a then-record federal deficit. (Ironically, Hoover's deficit budget would become a major point of attack for Roosevelt in the 1932 election.) He took the unprecedented step of federal relief for banks. In many ways, Hoover's policies formed a continuum, rather than a contrast, with Roosevelt's later approach.

But for all Hoover's innovations, the small federal government of his day could only give the economy a tiny push, far too weak to get the boulder of the economy rolling again. Perhaps in 1929 his measures might have helped, but in the much graver situation of 1931 and '32, they had no discernible impact. His natural lack of political finesse only worsened his problems, and he had increasing difficulty rallying Washington or Wall Street around any coherent plan. The public's views of him steadily hardened into hatred.

Roosevelt's Approach

In 1930, as the Depression worsened, Roosevelt was running for re-election in New York. (New York governors of the time served only two-year terms, though this would change to the modern four-year terms in 1938.) His Republican opponent—Charles H. Tuttle, a U.S. Attorney with a record of fighting corruption--resurrected concerns about Roosevelt's health and sought to link him to Tammany Hall. But Governor Roosevelt ran as if his opponent were Hoover, not Tuttle, criticizing the president's response to the Depression in every speech. He made retirement pensions and unemployment benefits the key themes of his campaign, and when Tuttle attacked, Roosevelt largely ignored him. Meanwhile, Eleanor went on a whirlwind speaking tour, speaking on her husband's behalf at hundreds of events.

The New York race drew intense national attention. In May, long-time Democratic Senator Burton K. Wheeler of Montana endorsed Roosevelt not only for governor in 1930 but for president in 1932. Hoover's Secretary of State Henry Stimson--a respected elder statesman that Roosevelt would later tap to head the U.S. war effort in World War II-- was dispatched to New York to campaign on

Tuttle's behalf and try to stop Roosevelt's momentum. This, too, had little effect.

Wow!

In the November elections, Democrats did well across the nation. They gained fifty-two seats in the House of Representatives and began the next session with a one-vote majority. Texan populist John Nance "Cactus Jack" Garner became the new Speaker of the House. Republicans also lost eight Senate seats, leaving the Senate divided 48-48 between the parties; Republicans maintained control of that chamber only through Vice President Charles Curtis's ability to break ties. But as usual, Roosevelt was running far ahead of his party. His closely watched race turned out to be a landslide. He won 1,770,342 votes to Tuttle's 1,045,341, more than double the margin of victory of any previous New York governor. Even areas considered solidly Republican opted for Roosevelt, and his support far exceeded the number of registered Democrats in the state.

The next morning, at Howe's orders but without consulting Roosevelt, his campaign manager James Farley appeared before the press to say the obvious: "I don't see how Mr. Roosevelt can escape becoming the next presidential nominee of his party."

The Fight for the Nomination

Despite Farley's words, despite Roosevelt's growing celebrity, despite the early endorsement of Senator Wheeler, Roosevelt's path to the nomination was still not assured. It was increasingly clear that the Democrats could win with almost any candidate in this election cycle; simply having a pulse and not being Herbert Hoover could catapult one into the White House. This made the 1932 nomination an even more valuable prize than usual.

Despite his 1928 defeat by Hoover--or perhaps because of it--Al Smith made it widely known that he hoped for a second nomination. Once a good friend, Smith had come to despise Roosevelt for the new governor's failure to let Smith continue to set policy. The maneuvering between their camps soon grew vicious. Roosevelt also faced a potential challenge from new Speaker of the House John Nance Garner.

For now, Roosevelt focused on governing New York, letting Howe and Farley take care of his national image. Farley made inroads with Democratic politicians in the West, while Howe recruited Woodrow Wilson's key advisor Edward House to build support in the South. In New York, Roosevelt constructed and dedicated a museum hall named for his now-deceased predecessor and cousin Theodore, subtly reminding voters of his connection to his revered relative.

He also continued his efforts to fight the Depression, proposing a "Temporary Emergency Relief Administration" (TERA) to provide jobs and necessities to the growing legions of unemployed. The agency would be overseen by Harry Hopkins, a workaholic social reformer who would be one of Roosevelt's key men for the rest of his life. In a testament to Roosevelt's growing political dominance in the state, the Republican legislature gave him first $20 million for this agency, then $30 million more, stipulating only that none of it be used for direct cash relief. Though the state's economic problems ran far too deep for such an easy fix, the program nonetheless proved popular.

The 1932 Democratic National Convention

Meanwhile, Al Smith continued to scheme for the nomination. He knew from the outset that he had no chance in beating Roosevelt in pledged delegates, but the Democratic convention rules required a two-thirds majority for the nomination. This was the rule that had blocked William McAdoo in 1920, and Smith himself in 1924, throwing the nomination to dark horse candidates. All Smith had to do was block Roosevelt or Garner from winning on the first ballot, and he could hope the convention might call on him as an elder statesman to break the impasse.

Roosevelt, in turn, focused on not making any mistakes that would hurt him in the general election. He refused to take a strong stance in the debate between internationalists and isolationists, allowing him to keep the support of both Wilsonians like House and arch-isolationists like Wheeler. Though his 1920 support of the League was on record, he implied he might or might not make the same decision today, a middle road that avoided confrontation with either side. Smith called for Roosevelt to take a stand on the repeal of Prohibition--an increasingly unpopular law--but Roosevelt demurred, not wishing to split the Southern vote.

On June 27, 1932, Roosevelt's campaign entered the Chicago-based convention just shy of the needed two-thirds of pledged delegates. His name was entered into nomination and seconded by Beulah Rebecca Hooks Hannah Tingley, the first time a female delegate addressed a Democratic National Convention. The first ballot came back with 666 votes for Roosevelt, 201 for Smith, and 90 for Garner.

Farley tried to reach out to Garner, whose delegates would put Roosevelt in reach of the needed 770, but Garner initially had the same hope as Smith. As John W. Davis had proved in 1924, if the convention deadlocked, absolutely anyone could be chosen. But after three ballots in which the numbers barely moved, Garner at last released his delegates to vote for others. Whether he did so out of party loyalty or in response to a direct promise of the vice presidency is still debated. (The convention would later vote him to this post unanimously, balancing the ticket between North and South.) On the fourth ballot, Roosevelt received 945 votes, making him the nominee.

No serious presidential candidate of the time attended the national conventions in person, and Roosevelt received the news of his nomination at the governor's mansion in Albany. On hearing the news, however, he took a doubly unprecedented step. He resolved to address the convention in person and to travel there by plane. Though air travel was increasingly common in America, politicians rarely used it, preferring to whistle-stop, and the fatal crash of Notre Dame coach Knute Rockne the year before had reminded the country of the dangers of commercial flight. To America, Roosevelt's flight symbolized the boldness of his leadership and his sense of urgency in battling the Depression.

Roosevelt's address to the convention set out a proud, liberal credo. Before a cheering crowd, he lambasted the Republican economic platform, which he said had brought prosperity only to a few: "But while they prate of economic laws, men and women are starving." Examined closely, his own proposals were riddled with contradictions; even as he promised unemployment relief and a greater government role in the economy, he attacked Hoover's federal budget as excessive and promised to cut spending. But his compassion and his urgency resonated with the desperate public, as did the phrase that defined his presidency for future generations: "I pledge you, I pledge myself, to a New Deal for the American people."

Campaign

After the success of the convention, Howe and Farley tried to dissuade Roosevelt from a national campaign. The presidency was clearly his to lose--why risk a gaffe for a few votes at a whistle-stop, or risk a collapse that might remind the public of his disability? But Roosevelt persisted, confident in his strength and wanting to bring his message before the American people face to face. He took to the rails, speaking across the country about electrical projects, unemployment relief, and aid to farmers. "Happy Days Are Here Again," his campaign's theme song, preceded and followed his speeches. Above all, he continued to hammer Hoover on the issue of federal spending, decrying the Republicans as irresponsible spendthrifts.

Hoover understandably developed a visceral hatred of Roosevelt, believing his rival to be a self-entitled aristocrat of weak character. Hoover believed that Roosevelt hadn't passed through anything like his own trials, conveniently forgetting Roosevelt's daily struggle with disability. He consequently did his best to ignore his challenger, pursuing what would later be called a Rose Garden strategy: ostentatiously doing the nation's business while his opponent campaigned and slung mud. But Hoover couldn't stay out of the dirt forever, and by September, he was openly accusing Roosevelt of encouraging class warfare and leading "the party of the mob." By this point, Hoover required massive police protection just to appear in public without being attacked by the mob he decried. Roosevelt kept the pressure on, determined not merely to win but to enter with a massive mandate.

He got it. On November 8, 1932, Roosevelt carried 42 of 48 states, and exceeded Hoover's vote tally by more than seven million votes. At last the Democrats were on the winning end of a landslide. Down-ticket candidates fared almost as well, and the Democrats would enter the next Congress with solid majorities in both houses. In March, Roosevelt would have the political support for almost any legislation he wanted, but for now he could only watch and wait. Under the laws of the day, Hoover would first serve as a lame duck for four more months, as the economy continued to crumble.

Chapter 5: Fighting for the Nation

Lame Duck Months

In March 1932--eight months before Roosevelt's election--Congress passed what would become the Twentieth Amendment to the United States Constitution, the so-called "Lame Duck Amendment." In the eighteenth century, the four-month interregnum between the presidential election and the inauguration had done no harm. In fact, it was a necessity: the slow communications and transportation of the time meant that an incoming president might well need four months to arrange a move to the capital and arrange his cabinet.

But by the nineteenth century, these lame duck months became an obvious problem. Abraham Lincoln suffered the worst, watching Southern state after Southern state declare for secession while President James Buchanan did nothing. By the time Lincoln was finally allowed to assume office, the situation was far worse than at the time of his election.

So in March 1932, the U.S. Congress finally took action, proposing a constitutional amendment to move presidential inaugurations to January 20. Some states quickly ratified the amendment, Virginia being the first. Within a month, 9 states of the required 36 had ratified, but then the momentum slowed to a crawl. Only 14 states had ratified by August, and on the day Roosevelt became the president-elect, only 17 states in total had ratified the amendment. Though the agonizing months between Hoover and Roosevelt persuaded every remaining state of the Union to ratify (Florida being the last, in March 1933), the change came too late to help Roosevelt's cause. (In fact, because of Roosevelt's long tenure and Truman's ascent to the office via Roosevelt's death, it would be a full twenty years before a president would actually take office sooner because of the amendment, Dwight D. Eisenhower in 1953). In 1933, Roosevelt would assume office on March 4 like every president before him.

During these months, Hoover continued to flounder, and Roosevelt was in no mood to help him. His political calculus was brutal but realistic. Hoover and Roosevelt both knew that a key step to recovery would be the cancellation of European war debts. Every economist said as much, though this would be more unpopular than ever with the panicking American people. Hoover wanted Roosevelt to make a joint statement with him favoring cancellation, but Roosevelt saw this as a pointless exercise--why waste political capital to help Hoover for something that would happen anyway?

What Roosevelt grasped, and Hoover did not, was that the American people's crisis of confidence needed political solutions, not just financial ones. Regardless of whether Roosevelt's policies were new or merely appeared to be new, the sense of a fresh start would itself provide a boost to consumer confidence, and therefore to the economy generally. Any sense that Roosevelt was coordinating with Hoover or continuing his policies would undercut this vital impression. Hoover also sought a public pledge that Roosevelt would maintain the gold standard and other elements of the Republican economic platform. Roosevelt, of course, rejected these requests out of hand.

It's surely also a factor that just as Hoover hated Roosevelt, Roosevelt personally hated Hoover. At a White House conference for governors in April 1932, Hoover kept Roosevelt waiting for more than an hour in a receiving line; Roosevelt's disability and braces made such a wait a painful misery. Biographers have never been sure whether Hoover did this intentionally--most likely he did not--but Roosevelt believed it to be a deliberate attempt to humiliate him. When the two met face to face following the November election, Hoover's smug condescension to his successor made Roosevelt dislike him more than ever.

A mixture of political considerations, policy differences, and raw personal dislike therefore kept Hoover and Roosevelt apart during these crucial months, even as a new wave of bank failures spread like wildfire. (By the time Roosevelt took office, scarcely a bank in America was confident in its solvency.)

Wow!

The Assassin

Giuseppe Zangara was a thirty-two-year-old Miami bricklayer who had immigrated from Italy three years before. Now he was unemployed, ill and in pain, and apparently suffering from increasing delusions. As he later described his motives to the Miami police: ""I have the gun in my hand. I kill kings and presidents first and next all capitalists." He claimed to have tried to kill the king of Italy before emigrating, but had never found the opportunity. He had considered killing Hoover, but had never mustered the resources for the trip north. In 1933, though, he learned that President-elect Roosevelt would be coming to him. Zangara, and the .32-caliber pistol he had just purchased, would be waiting.

On February 15, 1933, he shadowed the president's entourage throughout the day, waiting for his chance to strike. At last

Roosevelt stopped to give an impromptu speech from the back of an open car. Zangara stood atop a chair, raised his gun, and fired five shots.

But luck, as usual, favored Roosevelt. Zangara's chair was unstable, and an alert woman beside him struck him just as he fired. Zangara's bullets hit one of Roosevelt's bodyguards, two members of the audience, a CEO's wife in Roosevelt's entourage, and the Mayor of Chicago, Anthony Cermak, who was traveling beside Roosevelt to make amends for his support of Al Smith at the Democratic National Convention. Cermak died of complications from the wound a month later, but every shot missed the president-elect.

As he would on other occasions, Roosevelt demonstrated that his unflappable good humor concealed nerves of steel. He countermanded the Secret Service's orders to whisk him from the scene, insisting that medical attention for Cermak and the other wounded was the top priority. That evening with his staff, they were amazed to find him unrattled, his usual calm self. Franklin remembered that his cousin Theodore had once been shot in the chest by a Milwaukee saloonkeeper; the man had claimed that the ghost of William McKinley had ordered the assassination. Before he accepted medical attention, Theodore had delivered a scheduled ninety-minute speech while still bleeding. Now Franklin, too, had survived one of the darkest rites of passage of American presidents. His calm response to the incident added further to his public image in the month before he assumed office.

The Cabinet

Because of Roosevelt's four terms in office, his cabinet looms unusually large in American history. His long-time New York ally Frances Perkins, for example, not only became the first woman to serve in the Cabinet, but still holds the record as the longest-serving woman and the longest-serving Secretary of Labor (1933-45). Cordell Hull, an idealistic Tennessee Senator who helped secure the South for Roosevelt, became Secretary of State for a record-setting 11 years; in 1945, he would win the Nobel Peace Prize for his role in the founding of the United Nations. The temperamental Harold Ickes was named Secretary of the Interior, and his decade-plus in the office would shape a generation of national parks. Iowa progressive Henry A. Wallace, who would become an infamous apologist for Stalin and communism during Truman's presidency, was named Secretary of Agriculture.

A less successful appointment was Utah Governor George Dern, who was tapped to head the War Department. This was purely a political reward, bestowed for Dern's help in Roosevelt's run for the nomination. But Dern's lack of military expertise hardly seemed important; like Wilson before him, Roosevelt assumed his presidency would focus primarily on domestic concerns and have little need of war preparations. As for the Justice Department, Roosevelt's first choice as attorney general had a heart attack while traveling to the inauguration; his uninspiring successor, Homer S. Cummings, is known today mostly for supporting Roosevelt's later court-packing plan. Roosevelt's campaign manager Jim Farley was rewarded with the Postmaster Generalship, allowing him to distribute patronage nationally.

In terms of staff, Roosevelt was followed by his New York loyalists. Missy LeHand, his longtime secretary and possible lover, now became gatekeeper to the Oval Office. She would later be profiled in Newsweek as a "Super-Secretary" [Missy LeHand], and future Supreme Court Justice Felix Frankfurter described her as "the fifth most powerful person in the country." LeHand served Roosevelt until incapacitated by a 1941 stroke, after which she was succeeded by her assistant Grace Tully.

Steve Early continued to serve as press secretary, and Louis Howe remained on hand to give political counsel. Howe called himself Roosevelt's "no-man": when the president became carried away with a bad or risky idea, Howe would quickly throw cold water on it before he discussed it with other staff or made it public. But Howe began to suffer heart problems, likely related to his compulsive smoking, and by 1934 played a negligible role in policy-making. He died in 1936 and was given a state funeral by Roosevelt. Some biographers have speculated that if Howe had lived, Roosevelt might have been dissuaded from the 1937 court-packing debacle; it was the sort of foolishness that Howe specialized in squelching.

Roosevelt also founded his "Brain Trust" (sarcastically named by Howe), an elite collection of advisors with whom he debated economic policy long into the night. Roosevelt was no scholar and rarely read books or reports, but he loved to talk, and he had a remarkable capacity to absorb ideas from conversation. The first "Brain Trust" included Roosevelt stalwarts like Harry Hopkins, Frances Perkins, and Harold Ickes, joined by Columbia law professors Raymond Moley, Rexford Tugwell, and Adolf Berle, and future Supreme Court Justice Felix Frankfurter.

Reluctant First Lady

Eleanor's role in the new administration was less defined. For a decade now, she had served as Franklin's liaison to women's groups and other civic organizations. But Eleanor was surprisingly depressed by her husband's becoming president. Though this had been the goal throughout their married life, she feared Franklin's new duties would mean the end of the unusual partnership they had forged, a partnership that had given her a new sense of purpose throughout the past decade.

Most of all, Eleanor feared that she would lose her ability to be a political activist and volunteer leader; previous first ladies, like Lou Henry Hoover, had defined themselves strictly as society hostesses. (This is not to say that their role was trivial; the convivial Lou Henry Hoover, for example, played a vital role in her husband's administration by smoothing over the friction created by her husband's glacial reserve.) Eleanor was so upset that she even considered divorcing her husband on the eve of his inauguration. The journalist Lorena

Hickok, a confidant and possible lover of Eleanor's, would later subtitle her biography "Reluctant First Lady."

But as it turned out, Eleanor needn't have worried. She would ultimately prove even more useful to Franklin, and to the country, as First Lady than she had before. The public never learned of Eleanor's depression, and Howe and Hickok soon encouraged her to find satisfaction by redefining the role of First Lady as she pleased.

Lorena Hickok's presence itself may have been a help. At the time of Franklin's inauguration, Hickok had become the nation's best-known, and best-paid, female reporter, the first ever to work for the Associated Press. Assigned to cover Eleanor during the presidential election, Hickok struck up a close friendship, and as time progressed, possibly something more.

The exact nature of this relationship continues to be debated by biographers, and likely will be debated forever--the existing evidence is suggestive but not quite conclusive. (Hickok was an open lesbian, or at least as open as one could be in 1932 America.) At a minimum, Eleanor could be said to have had a "schoolgirl crush" on Hickok. The pair openly professed love for each other; Eleanor kept a picture of Hickok on her desk and wrote Hickok that she kissed the picture every morning and every night in Hickok's absence. <u>The couple exchanged more than 3,000 letters in their lifetimes,</u> a small number of which Hickok later destroyed rather than turn over to historians. When apart, they wrote one another of their longing to be together again and lie down together in each others' arms. But as biographer Doris Kearns Goodwin observes, the obsession of modern historians with what precisely the couple did while lying down together is a bit beside the point.

Eleanor had found a deep, loving relationship, whether it consisted of friendly embraces or something more.

This relationship carried Eleanor through the difficult early transition to the White House, but as Franklin's presidency progressed, Eleanor and Hickok gradually drew apart. Whatever Eleanor's intentions, Hickok was hopelessly in love and always wanted more from Eleanor: more attention, more time, more affection. At the same time, Eleanor characteristically took on more and more responsibilities and commitments as First Lady. Some friction was inevitable, and by 1937, the women were much less close.

Hickok was not Eleanor's only emotional affair. Eleanor also had a long-running and difficult-to-define relationship with a man named Earl Miller, a New York State Trooper assigned to Franklin's detail when he was governor in 1929. Twelve years younger than Eleanor, Miller was affectionate, handsome, and athletic--he had even been a member of the 1920 American Olympic team. He taught Eleanor to ride and to swim, and had his own room in her New York apartment and her Hyde Park cottage, Val-Kill. <u>Friends wrote with alarm about the couple's unconcealed affection for one another in public places.</u>

As with Hickok's destruction of selected letters, the lack of documentary evidence about Eleanor and Miller's relationship is itself suggestive. The two wrote one another constantly for forty years, up until Eleanor's death, but not a single letter has been found by biographers. Miller was married and divorced three times; he frankly stated later that at least two of those marriages were meant to defuse gossip about himself and Eleanor. In his third divorce, his soon-to-be ex-wife threatened to name Eleanor as a co-respondent.

Franklin appeared unbothered by Eleanor's affairs, and even to support them. In the words of Jean Edward Smith:

Eleanor's friendship with Miller paralleled Franklin's relationship with Missy LeHand. Just as Missy provided FDR with the adoration and love his wife could not, so Miller made up for what Franklin could not give. Remarkably, both ER and Franklin recognized, accepted, and encouraged the arrangement. Missy and Earl became members of the family. Eleanor gave Missy the larger bedroom near FDR's in Albany while she took a smaller one down the hall, and Franklin was equally attentive to Earl's requirements. Eleanor and Franklin were strong-willed people who cared greatly for each other's happiness but realized their own inability to provide for it.

Just as Eleanor made her own path romantically, so too did she make her own path politically. She soon became controversial as the most activist First Lady to date, lobbying the government and her husband for women's rights and for racial equality. While Franklin and Eleanor occasionally clashed on these issues, Eleanor also provided her husband useful political cover on the left: she could reach out to African American groups in a way he could not without losing the support of Southern senators. Eleanor set new precedents in every area--no First Lady had ever before had a newspaper column, held a press conference of her own, or address a national political convention--and redefined her office even more than her husband would redefine his.

The Hundred Days: Saving the Banks

With the banking crisis at its peak, Franklin Roosevelt entered office with the nation in a state of emergency. He used powers from the Trading with the Enemy Act to declare a banking holiday, stanching any further bleeding, and he immediately ordered a special session of Congress. Four days later, Democrats rammed through the Emergency Banking Act, expanding the powers of the president and Federal Reserve Board to infuse cash into the nation's financial sector. The Federal Reserve Board announced that it would publish the names of depositors who had withdrawn large amounts of money or gold, a measure designed to shame citizens back to the banks. The night before the banks reopened, Roosevelt gave his first presidential Fireside Chat, promising the nation that their cash would be safe in the newly supervised banking system.

The results were tremendous. When the banks nervously reopened on March 13, not only were the "runs" at an end, but people were lining up to deposit their money. Rallying at the news, stock prices rose by 15% in a single day. One of the most frightening aspects of the Great Depression was already over, and Roosevelt had only been in office for nine days.

It would be one of his finest moments throughout the Depression and starkly demonstrated his gifts. Whereas Hoover had battered the nation with theories and statistics and seen no results, Roosevelt's political deftness and natural showmanship allowed him to reassure the skittish public. Once the public had recognized their true enemy as "fear itself," they were ready to head back to the banks. The columnist Walter Lippmann had offered a famously withering critique of Roosevelt during the campaign, summing him up as "a pleasant man who, without any important qualifications for the office, would very much like to be President." Now Lippmann wrote approvingly that "in one week, the nation, which had lost confidence in everything and everybody, has regained confidence in the government and in itself."

The Hundred Days: Saving the Farmers

The rest of the Hundred Days would be more of a mixed bag, but in a way, that was how Roosevelt intended it. He was not a systematic thinker, but a pragmatic one, and his lack of ideology proved an asset as the nation sailed into uncharted economic waters. He conceived of his New Deal as a long-running experiment in macroeconomics, telling his staff: "Take a method and try it. If it fails, try another. But above all, try something."

Roosevelt offered some early sops to the right. He proposed and passed a bill reducing the salaries of government workers and (surprising in light of the recent "Bonus Army" fiasco) the pensions of U.S. Army veterans. He created the Civilian Conservation Corps, which required poor youth to take jobs on new projects in the National Parks and send most of their wages home to their families. Though initially criticized by progressives as "forced labor," the program lasted for ten years, employing more than three million young men and women and reshaping federal lands on a scale previously undreamed of. Roosevelt also successfully overturned the Volstead Act, fulfilling a bipartisan effort to end Prohibition. He insisted on a balanced federal budget, though he managed this trick only by adding funds from an "emergency budget" onto the supposedly balanced regular budget.

But he also departed from the gold standard, creating near-hysteria among conservatives. With the virtue of hindsight, we can easily see today that a currency does not need the gold standard to survive, but this was far from clear at the time. Republicans denounced him, as did Roosevelt's persistent gadfly Al Smith, even as the savvier titans of Wall Street quietly applauded.

But Roosevelt got no such right-wing applause when he created the Federal Emergency Relief Administration, which distributed federal funds to state governments for unemployment relief. Roosevelt was now approaching the line that Hoover had drawn so starkly: direct federal relief for the unemployed. Harry Hopkins would be given control of this new agency.

The Agricultural Adjustment Act (AAA) took things even further. Brain Truster Rexford Tugwell had persuaded Roosevelt that "overproduction" was a key cause of the Great Depression--that technology had caused the American economy to reach a final plateau of production, and that the only solution was for every American to work fewer hours to spread the remaining work around. Though this idea is ridiculed by economists today, macroeconomics was in its infancy in the 1930s, and the proposal was widely popular. Related petitions circulated for 30-hour work weeks and for early forced retirement of older workers.

Luckily for the nation, the only real legacy of these proposals was farm subsidies. Farmers were among the worst hit by the Great

Depression. (The Dust Bowl (erosion caused by over-farming and severe drought) in the West had uprooted tens of thousands of families, making it one of the worst manmade environmental disasters until Chernobyl and anthropogenic climate change.) Falling consumer demand caused by the Depression made things unimaginably worse. The average farmer's income fell by more than two-thirds between 1929 and 1932.

Applying Tugwell's ideas, Roosevelt and his Brain Trust blamed overproduction, which they believed glutted the market and drove down prices. The AAA proposed a system in which farmers would be subsidized to leave fields fallow. As part of the initial implementation, Secretary of Agriculture Henry Wallace even paid farmers to kill millions of hogs and destroy millions of acres of cotton already growing in the fields. In the words of David M. Kennedy, the American agricultural sector thereafter became "a virtual ward of the state," which it remains to the present day. Though the bill was designed to help small farmers the most, it quickly became clear that most of its funds would be claimed by larger agricultural companies.

The Hundred Days: Saving Labor

The most famous New Deal creation, the National Recovery Administration (NRA), also soon saw most of its funds diverted to business interests. Designed to inject stimulus money into the economy through public works, the NRA failed in this goal when Roosevelt put Secretary of the Interior Harold Ickes in charge of the related Public Works Administration (PWA). Ickes obsessed over the minutiae of each project, and released funds only at a trickle. The NRA was left to try to coordinate prices and production among businesses, which Wall Street called socialism and labor called price-fixing.

When the Supreme Court struck down the act establishing the NRA as unconstitutional, Roosevelt was in some ways relieved. Though initially widely praised, the NRA had quickly become a public relations nightmare. He took the funds Ickes had failed to distribute and turned them over to Hopkins as a new agency, the CWA (Civil Works Administration).

But the NRA was far from a total failure. Like many of Roosevelt's economic efforts, the symbolism itself made a difference, and workers were thrilled to see a president seemingly on their side. Historian William Manchester compares it to "a spectacularly successful football rally followed by a lost game." And even after the Supreme Court decision, parts of the NRA's labor codes were reincorporated by Congress into the National Labor Relations Act of 1935. Child labor was banned, and for the first time, collective bargaining was recognized as a right of workers in most industries.

The Hundred Days Assessed

It's hard to overstate the importance in American history of Roosevelt's Hundred Days. Congress set an all-time record for legislative activity, and many of laws they passed are still with us. Prohibition was overturned; the banks were saved; federal deposit insurance was created; American farmers would be subsidized for decades to come; child labor was banned; unprecedented amounts of federal construction began. Unions were officially recognized, and soon swelled into a major political force. The Glass-Steagall Act was signed into law, separating commercial and investment banking and guaranteeing that America would not suffer another depression caused by bank failures-- previously a regular occurrence--until its 1999 repeal. The Tennessee Valley Authority was established, putting the federal government in the business of building dams and bringing electricity into rural areas in an unprecedented way.

But most of all, the Hundred Days changed the way Americans thought about their government, and about each other. Hoover had bluntly argued that the federal government did not exist to help those in need, and that direct aid only fostered dependence. Roosevelt, in turn, argued that the government was only the representative of the people, and the people should help one another in crisis through this representative. The argument has echoed for more than eight decades since, but it is an argument that really began in the Roosevelt years.

The Hundred Days also reshaped the presidency, for better and for worse. Coolidge and Hoover had seen themselves as administrators, and Coolidge in particular went out of his way to take as little presidential action as possible. Roosevelt saw himself as a leader, the captain in a storm. This was the beginning of the so-called "Imperial Presidency" that continued throughout the century, allowing strong leadership in wartime, but arguably also excesses like the Vietnam War and Watergate. Only a hundred days into the 1,502 he would spend as president, it was already clear that after FDR, nothing would be the same.

Backlash: The Left

Despite some initial successes, Roosevelt's New Deal was not a panacea for the Great Depression. Unemployment remained shockingly high, the farmers shockingly desperate. Leaders of black Americans protested that the largesse of the New Deal had so far been distributed almost entirely to whites. (As Ira Katznelson details in When Affirmative Action Was For Whites, this charge was sadly accurate.) While he remained generally popular, Roosevelt found himself under pressure on all sides.

One threat that Roosevelt took very seriously was Huey "Kingfish" Long, a populist senator from Louisiana who ran on the slogan "every man a king, but no man wears the crown." Born dirt poor, Long rose to political prominence by attacking the out-of-state oil corporations that dominated Louisiana politics before him. When he was elected governor, he taxed the oilmen like mad to pay for public works in his backwater state, bullied every state and county official into his camp, and soon took literally dictatorial power for himself. In one instance, he even marched on

New Orleans with state militia when the city government disobeyed him.

By 1934, he was in the U.S. Senate, and despite his early support of Roosevelt's program, he soon saw the chance to attack the president from the left. He launched a campaign to seize and redistribute every large fortune in America, and his Share Our Wealth Society, claimed a membership of more than 5 million. Speaking to a group of fellow senators in private, he predicted that someday soon the American people would storm the building to hang them all, and Long himself would be leading the charge. Roosevelt described him as "the second most dangerous man in America"--second only to General Douglas MacArthur, who had attacked the "Bonus Army" and already made his contempt for civilian leadership crystal clear. Long would remain a threat on Roosevelt's left until the senator's September 1935 assassination.

Roosevelt was also sharply criticized by his onetime ally Father Charles Coughlin, the then-famous "radio priest." A Detroit-based Roman Catholic priest, Coughlin took his populist oratory to the airwaves every week. At first he had supported Roosevelt's New Deal, but by 1934 found it too conservative. Coughlin then turned on his former favorite with incredible vehemence. He railed at Roosevelt as an ally of Wall Street bankers, called him the "anti-God", and openly suggested he should be assassinated. He increasingly, and obsessively, warned of a conspiracy of Jewish financiers lurking behind Wall Street and the president. His magazine began to reprint parts of the famous anti-Semitic forgery, The Protocols of the Elders of Zion, and by the end of the decade, he was open in his admiration for Hitler and Mussolini. Though the Vatican had long tried to silence him, it was World War II that finally gave Roosevelt the excuse to ban Coughlin from the radio as an enemy propagandist.

A third challenge on Roosevelt's left came from the socialist author Upton Sinclair, best known for his 1906 novel The Jungle, which exposed the horrors that immigrant workers faced in Chicago's meatpacking industry. (Predictably, readers reacted most strongly not to the plight of the impoverished workers, but to Sinclair's revelations about the poor hygiene and quality of the plants' meat; within a year, the federal government responded by passing new regulations and creating inspectors who would eventually become the Food and Drug Administration.) In 1934, Sinclair won the Democratic primary for the California governorship with a pledge to entirely abolish private property. Horrified, Roosevelt evaded Sinclair's requests for an endorsement, and Sinclair was soundly defeated by his Republican opponent.

Backlash: The Right

The Republicans were even more critical of the New Deal than were Roosevelt's leftist opponents. They needed time to recover from the shellacking of the 1932 election and the terror of the 1932-33 banking crisis, of course. But after a breather, they jumped back into the ring swinging.

Hoover continued to criticize his successor for curtailing American freedom, and began to push for a Constitutional amendment giving more power back to the states. Republican criticisms were joined by a surprising number of conservative Democrats, including the past two presidential nominees, Al Smith and John W. Davis. The embittered Smith was particularly virulent, accusing Roosevelt of seeking to become a dictator, of owing his real allegiance to Moscow, and of wanting to replace the national anthem with the

Communist "Internationale." Businessmen also became increasingly hostile, and in 1935 the U.S. Chamber of Commerce began open attacks on Roosevelt's policies.

In an indication of the schizophrenic politics of Roosevelt's day, he also faced Republicans threatening to run on his left. Robert La Follette--the progressive Wisconsin Republican who had made a doomed 1924 independent bid for the presidency-- grumbled increasingly about Roosevelt's policy. The Democratic Burton K. Wheeler, who had been La Follette's running mate, and later so notably endorsed FDR in 1930, openly called for a third party challenge to the president. La Follette's son Philip heeded the call and re-formed the Progressive Party, peeling away some left-wing Republicans.

When the 1934 Congressional midterm elections arrived, the Republicans thought they had their moment to strike. Roosevelt thought so, too. When James Farley told the president he thought they could break even in both houses, Roosevelt dismissed it as wishful thinking. But 1934 bucked the trend for midterm elections; the Democrats gained several seats in both houses and also picked up several governorships, making the Republicans more irrelevant than ever.

The Second New Deal

With a fresh mandate, Roosevelt's Brain Trust went back to work. The legislation later known as the "Second New Deal" also failed to stop the Great Depression, but it, too, would become a permanent part of American life.

The centerpiece was the Social Security Act. This act provided direct aid to widows, orphans, and the unemployed, but its most notable feature was guaranteed income for elderly citizens. Unlike similar European systems, the act was self-financing, supported by a payroll tax. Roosevelt later commented that the tax was a political necessity, not a financial one: "We put those payroll taxes there so as to give the contributors a legal, moral, and political right to collect their pensions and their unemployment benefits. With those taxes in there, no damn politician can ever scrap my social security program."

It's unlikely that this program helped fight the Great Depression in the short run; in fact, it likely prolonged it slightly, since by collecting for future retirement, the government was taking money out of the economy rather than adding money in--the opposite of a stimulus. But Social Security became a fixed part of American life over the next century, and many Americans have come to see providing for elderly citizens as a basic duty of the federal government. Roosevelt considered this bill to be the most important of his presidency.

In 1935, Democrats also passed legislation creating the Works Progress Administration. The WPA, overseen primarily by the ubiquitous Harry Hopkins, provided 3 million jobs in its first year alone and by 1936 employed 7% of the American work force. These jobs were often distributed through local governments and local party bosses, and Republicans derided it as Tammany Hall-style patronage on a national scale. There was some justice to this, and Congress eventually removed this aspect with the 1939 Hatch Act.

But the WPA also built 572,000 miles of highway, and innumerable schools, parks, and hospitals across the country, as well financing budding artists in all fields like Orson Welles, Burt Lancaster, Jackson Pollack, Willem de Kooning, Saul Bellow, Zora Neale Hurston,

Ralph Ellison, John Steinbeck, and Richard Wright. Some of these artists proved their own worst enemies, and their critiques of capitalism and America itself led to most of the arts funding being cut. But the WPA as a whole would provide 8 million jobs during the Depression, and would only be dismantled in 1943 when World War II brought about such low unemployment that the program was no longer needed.

Roosevelt vs. the Supreme Court

During Roosevelt's first term of office, he faced a Supreme Court headed by Charles Evans Hughes, the 1916 Republican challenger against Woodrow Wilson. The war between Roosevelt and the Court began in earnest when the NRA was struck down in a unanimous opinion on May 27, 1935. Hughes castigated the law in unusually harsh terms; Roosevelt retaliated by comparing the court's decision to the infamous Dred Scott ruling, which had upheld slavery throughout the United States and banned African Americans from citizenship.

The Supreme Court was undeterred, and more legislation rapidly fell. The court invalidated the farm subsidies of the AAA. They banned the new Securities and Exchange Commission as an abuse of government authority. They banned both federal and state governments from setting minimum wages. They even banned the federal government from working with states to ensure the solvency of banks. According to William Manchester, where the Supreme Court had previously struck down only 60 laws in 140 years, they now invalidated 11 of Roosevelt's laws in a single year.

Part of the problem was certainly the liberal nature of the laws, and their radical reimagining of the relationship between citizens and government. But as Jean Edward Smith points out, another part of the problem was how hastily and broadly these new laws had been written, with almost no attention to Constitutional precedent. The fact that many of these laws would later be upheld when more carefully drafted indicates that the Hughes Court was not implacably opposed to their content.

Regardless of the cause, Roosevelt's anger at the Court's actions would lead him to the greatest overreach of his political career. His instincts had not abandoned him yet, though. He knew that in some ways the justices had given him a gift: perfect fodder for the '36 campaign trail.

Roosevelt in '36

After the landslide of '32 and the midterm victory of '34, it's surprising to read how many political commentators of the day predicted Roosevelt would be a one-term president. The newspapers in particular, most of which had conservative ownership, were arrayed heavily against him. But Roosevelt had sidestepped print media with his Fireside Chats, and was confident in his ability to take the issues directly to the people.

The Republicans faced a dilemma in 1936. Given the popularity of so much of Roosevelt's platform, they couldn't outright oppose the New Deal and hope to win, but neither did they wish to betray their core principles. Like so many political parties before and since, they settled for having the worst of both worlds. After a sad episode in which Herbert Hoover attempted to secure his third nomination in a row--he was greeted with applause but no votes whatsoever--the convention settled on Alfred "Alf" Landon, the bland governor of Kansas. Despite being nicknamed the "Kansas Coolidge," Landon had voted for La Follette, not Coolidge, in 1924, and had impressive progressive credentials, including openly supporting some redistribution of private property. He didn't want to reverse Roosevelt's policies, but to carry them on more effectively. But he preferred to play the statesman and let other party figures get in the political mud with the Democrats; his advocates were so conservative in their arguments that the country had little chance to notice that Landon was as progressive as FDR.

Roosevelt, meanwhile, attacked big business with new vigor. Until now, he had tried to keep a semblance of good relations with the business community, but the bridges were finally burned and he had nothing left to lose. In his acceptance speech at the 1936 Democratic National Convention, he declared, "I should like it to be said of my first administration that in it the forces of selfishness and of lust for power have met their match. I should like to have it said of my second administration that in it these forces met their master."

Despite feeling increasingly confident, Roosevelt again campaigned hard around the nation, seeking to build another mandate. In the end, Landon carried only Maine and Vermont, losing even his home state of Kansas. Roosevelt won 61% of the popular vote, a record beaten in all of American history only by Lyndon Johnson in 1964. The election was also notable for being the first in which more African Americans voted for Democrats than for Republicans; the New Deal was welcome help to this most desperate segment of

America's population, no matter how unfairly distributed--and no matter how little Roosevelt himself had yet to do for civil rights.

Overreach

Historians have noted that a massive second-term mandate often leads a president directly to folly. It happened to Thomas Jefferson, who followed his wildly successful first term (the Barbary War, the Louisiana Purchase, Lewis and Clark) with the debacle of his second (the Burr trial, the Embargo Act). It happened to Lyndon Johnson, who followed the success of his brief first term, in which he passed the 1964 Civil Rights Act, by leading the country into the Vietnam War.

And it happened to Franklin D. Roosevelt.

Now sworn in for his second term, with the people freshly at his back, Roosevelt was determined that the Supreme Court not be allowed to dismantle the entire New Deal. Beyond preserving his political legacy, he believed that the justices were putting the entire country at risk by blocking economic recovery and the people's will. The Supreme Court had jumped to the forefront of political controversies before, as with John Marshall's opposition to Jefferson, the Dred Scott decision, or the Supreme Court's attempt to stop Andrew Jackson from dispossessing the Cherokee of their lands. But Roosevelt was the first president to come fully up against what would become a uniquely American paralysis: a 9-member, unelected body whose members sit for life, and yet have the final say on all of America's most controversial issues, including campaign finance reform, segregation, government health care, gay marriage, gun control, abortion, affirmative action, and the death penalty.

In 1937, Roosevelt thought he had the solution. The number of justices on the Supreme Court is fixed by Congress, not the Constitution; if his congressional majority allowed him to appoint more justices, he could add as many as were needed to swing the Court his own way. But Roosevelt made a unusual political blunder in rolling out the plan. Overconfident in his new mandate, he hatched his plan in secret and failed to consult any congressional leaders before submitting the legislation.

His press conference, only two weeks after his second inauguration, therefore struck Washington like a thunderbolt, and congressmen were still reeling when they formally received his proposed bill minutes later. Roosevelt's vice president, John Nance Garner, immediately and openly opposed him. House Judiciary Chair Harron Sumners declared, "boys, here's where I cash in my chips," and refused to propose the bill to his committee. Burton K. Wheeler led both Republican and Democratic progressives and conservatives in full-fledged revolt. Southern conservatives were particularly alarmed at the prospect of a new, activist Supreme Court that might return the rights of African Americans that had been granted, and then lost, in the Reconstruction Era. Even Chief Justice Hughes broke with precedent by writing directly to the Senate to protest the plan, baldly stating that "this proposed bill would destroy the Court as an institution."

Roosevelt continued on the attack, confident that he enjoyed the public's support on the issue. But the press denounced him strenuously, comparing his actions to those of the fascist leaders seizing Europe, and fewer and fewer of his party came to his defense. Then in several narrow decisions, the Supreme Court upheld key parts of New Deal legislation on their current docket, including overturning one of their own year-old decisions: states could now pass minimum wage laws, they ruled. Cynics immediately called this "the switch in time that saved nine," but Hughes and other justices argued that the later legislation had been better drafted than the rushed bills of the Hundred Days. Whatever the case, the decisions rendered Roosevelt's court-packing plan a moot point.

Amazingly, Roosevelt still fought on. Even when Justice Van Devanter handed in his resignation, allowing FDR to appoint a justice of his own, he fought on. (Ultimately Roosevelt would appoint eight justices, one short of a complete court of his own.) Vice President Garner left for Texas rather than preside over this debate for Roosevelt, and still FDR fought on. Finally the Majority Leader of the Senate, Joe Robinson, dropped dead of a heart attack, surely exacerbated by the stress of trying to corral enough votes for

Roosevelt's plan. In an uncharacteristic act of political spite, Roosevelt--who blamed Robinson in part for the bill's delay--refused to go to the funeral, further poisoning his relations with the remaining senators. Only then, having squandered his entire mandate and split his party, did Roosevelt finally give up on his plan.

In just six months after one of the biggest landslides of American history, Roosevelt had made himself into a lame duck. And worse was still to come.

The Roosevelt Recession

While FDR fought his ill-advised battle for the Court, smaller battles were breaking out across the nation as newly-empowered unions began a series of sit-down strikes. These strikes gave the business community, and the conservative

Democrats with whom they allied, fresh cause to mistrust Roosevelt.

And then in May 1937, the economy began to backslide, the first significant slump of the Roosevelt presidency. Later historians have given various explanations for this downturn. Many New Deal projects had already peaked in their spending, Roosevelt was again trying to balance the budget, and Social Security taxes were now taking money out of the economy. The economy simply may not have yet recovered sufficiently to be taken off the life support of government stimulus to be withdrawn.

The 1937 recession may also have been a chance result of the normal boom-bust cycle, unrelated to any government policy. But having worked so hard to blame Hoover's policies for the 1932 Depression, Roosevelt was hard pressed to explain why his own policies should not be held responsible for the current downturn. Somewhat implausibly, he blamed a deliberate conspiracy of big business to withdraw capital in order to sabotage the economy and sink his presidency, but this argument gained little traction. Alliterative critics soon dubbed the downturn the "Roosevelt Recession."

Roosevelt saw the 1938 elections as a chance to reclaim his mandate as well as his leadership of the party. This time Roosevelt felt he must not only maintain the Democratic majority in Congress, but purge the Southern conservative Democrats who were increasingly arrayed against him.

The 1937 legislative session saw a major fight over an Anti-Lynching Bill, the only civil rights measure the federal government had considered in some time. Though the bill was virtually toothless, Southern senators could tolerate no interference in their sovereign right to terrorize black citizens. Roosevelt refused to participate, knowing he would lose an entire wing of his party if he did so. (Later Democrats would face the same problem; when Lyndon Johnson finally passed civil rights legislation in 1964 and 1965, the South shifted overnight from largely voting Democratic to largely voting Republican, and has remained that way ever since.)

But Roosevelt hoped to undermine the Southern bloc one contest at a time, and in the 1938 primary season, he inserted himself into Senate races in Georgia, South Carolina, and Maryland. In each case, the conservative Democrat handily beat Roosevelt's handpicked replacement. Roosevelt had only split the party further, and the Republicans took full advantage, winning 13 new governorships and nearly taking back the House and Senate.

As 1939 began and he finally, reluctantly, turned his full attention to the world stage, Roosevelt had fewer friends in Washington to help him than ever before.

Assessing the New Deal

Historians generally agree that the New Deal was at best a limited success as a recovery program. The Great Depression really ended only with the massive government spending of World War II and the countless jobs it created. At least some of Roosevelt's ideas, such as deliberately suppressing production, are in retrospect foolish or even disastrous. Some conservative historians, such as the British author Paul Johnson, have argued that Roosevelt and even Hoover's attempts at stimulus and intervention actually prolonged the Depression, which would otherwise have been just a brief downturn in the usual boom-bust cycle.

Other historians have argued that Roosevelt was groping in the right direction, but simply failed to go far enough. In 1938, he at last explicitly embraced deficit spending--the idea that the government would borrow when the economy was weak to pump money back into the economy. But it was a classic case of too little, too late. The U.S. economy was worth $100 billion at the time, and after eight years of economic carnage, Roosevelt proposed to add just $3 billion more.

It's useful to contrast this with the 2008-09 financial crisis, when Presidents George W. Bush and Barack Obama between them made a swift injection of almost a trillion dollars of stimulus into a seventeen-trillion dollar economy. Though this stimulus was offset by an almost equal drop in state government spending, a recent poll found that more than 80% of economists agree that unemployment would have been much worse without the compensatory federal spending.

In this school of thought, Roosevelt was on the right track, but failed to pursue it far enough both due to political pressures (his previous promises on balancing the budget, opposition of conservatives) and his own economic prejudices. The New Deal provided relief for the unemployed, but no long-term jobs.

But as David M. Kennedy points out, even if it failed in its stated goal of ending the Great Depression, the New Deal restructured the American economy for the better in fundamental ways. Social Security provided the start of a basic social safety net. The Securities and Exchange Commission cracked down on Wall Street corruption, allowing smaller investors to enter the market at much less risk of being swindled. Federal deposit insurance guaranteed that there would be no more bank runs in America's future. Switching from a fixed to a floating currency freed the economy for future growth. The end of Prohibition reduced local, state, and federal corruption and returned alcohol taxes to state treasuries. The legalization of collective bargaining allowed working-class and middle-class Americans a greater share of company profits. Any one of these would have been a major accomplishment for any president; by passing them all, Roosevelt set the stage for an economic post-war boom that would be among the greatest in world history. Historians who believe Roosevelt's New Deal fatally undermined the U.S. economy have to tie themselves in knots explaining why just two years after his death, with all these policies still in place, that same economy began to grow at a record-shattering pace.

Throughout Roosevelt's political career, there were conservative and business interests who accused him of trying to institute socialism or communism in America. Roosevelt was always puzzled and frustrated by this charge. His policies had never transferred the means of production to government--the fundamental tenet of socialism--and he openly opposed those like Upton Sinclair and Huey Long who did call for such measures. Without Roosevelt's vigorous experiments and reassurance of the public, the country could plausibly have followed such left-wing demagogues, or a MacArthur-like reactionary from the right. This was happening to democracies all across Europe. Roosevelt saw himself not as an enemy to capitalism, but the best friend the free markets ever had: the man who saved capitalism from itself.

Chapter 6:
Fighting for the World

The Long Road to War: Europe

Even as the Great Depression consumed America, another, greater threat lurked on the horizon. Few American observers paid real attention, and fewer still raised any significant alarms. But the rise of fascist governments in Germany, Italy, Hungary, and Japan were not the distant problems they seemed, but crises that would cause 400,000 American deaths before they had run their course.

Like the Great Depression, the Second World War had its roots in the first. Because Allied soldiers had never properly invaded Germany in World War I--rather, they had annihilated the German Army in France--German citizens never tasted real defeat. Military figures such as Paul von Hindenburg and Erich Ludendorff carefully arranged that the civilian government, not the military, would sign the severe surrender terms, paving the way for the charge that civilian and Jewish elements had betrayed an otherwise successful German military--the "stab-in-the-back" myth. The German people therefore never accepted war reparations payments as justified, leading to an endless series of international crises until the debt was finally annulled, unpaid.

And then Adolf Hitler, a failed artist and wounded World War I veteran, stepped onto the scene. A skilled orator who pulled no punches in criticizing the Versailles Treaty, he rose to the top of the National Socialist (Nazi) hierarchy by 1921, and took his fervently nationalist, anti-Semitic message to the nation. In 1923, the Nazis attempted their first coup in the region of Bavaria, the so-called "Beer Hall Putsch." The putsch failed, but Hitler received only a light jail term, during which he wrote Mein Kampf. He continued to orate and organize after his release, but was viewed by most as a lunatic fringe element.

That began to change with the Great Depression. Desperate people look for desperate measures, and a minority to scapegoat is always welcome. Hitler found the nation newly receptive to his argument that shadowy cabals of Jewish financiers were undermining the German nation, and Nazi ranks began to swell. Germany's Communist Party grew at the same time, and each movement fed off the other in a strange symbiotic relationship; the communists called the Nazis capitalism's true face, while the Nazis began to persuade more reasonable conservative elements that Hitler was the only hope of stopping a Communist takeover. Hitler took second place in the presidential election of 1932, and the winner, Paul von Hindenburg, appointed him Chancellor to maintain the conservative coalition in 1933.

That year, a Dutch communist was arrested following a fire at the Reichstag building. Historians remain divided as to whether this was an individual attack, a wider plot by Communists, or a "false-flag" operation by the Nazis themselves. Whatever the case, the Nazis used the incident as a pretext to pass sweeping emergency decrees that effectively turned the democratic Weimar Republic into a dictatorship. The already-ineffectual Hindenburg died in 1934, and Hitler assumed his powers as well.

Having secured total control in Germany, Hitler turned his attention to the outside world. Despite Germany's military weakness, he reoccupied the Rhineland in 1936, an action his generals considered so foolish that they were prepared to overthrow him the moment the French mobilized against them. But the French mobilization never came.

Outside of Germany, the European public had been so sickened by the brutality of World War I that they felt another conflict must be avoided at all costs. Many also recalled the reluctance of Americans to join in World War I, and saw no reason to believe that they could rely on Roosevelt's government now. (Nor did Roosevelt, focused as he was on domestic affairs, give them any reason to think so.) The French government and British Prime Minister Neville Chamberlain pursued a doctrine of "appeasement" instead. Later, this word would be a synonym for diplomatic folly (or for some hardliners, for any diplomacy at all). At the time, however, it was a hugely popular choice, and the leaders who traded their neighbors for a few more years of peace were celebrated around the world.

Hitler seized Austria in a bloodless invasion called the Anschluss, and the heavily industrialized area of Czechoslovakia known as the Sudetenland. Britain and France once again ratified these seizures by treaty, the latter at Munich in 1938. Returning from Munich, Chamberlain proclaimed that he had avoided a war scare and brought "peace in our time," and was welcomed by the British people as a hero. Winston Churchill, an irascible former minister of several Liberal and Conservative governments, railed against the Munich pact, but found no real audience.

Hitler also found an ally in Benito Mussolini, the fascist dictator of Italy. Like Hitler, he had brought seeming order to democratic disorganization. Most famously, he had "made the trains run on time," claiming credit for improvements to Italy's train system actually instituted by a parliamentary committee before he took power. His followers, known as "blackshirts," violently suppressed opposition until the boisterous, clownish Mussolini ruled unopposed.

America followed these events with only passing interest. American Jewish groups were alarmed by the increasing mistreatment of their German brethren, particularly after the murderous Kristallnacht ("Night of Broken Glass") of November 9, 1938, when Jewish businesses were destroyed in nationwide rioting. But the casual anti-Semitism of 1930s America meant that the general public paid little notice; even in later wartime propaganda films, the fate of Germany's Jews would barely be mentioned. Despite frantic behind-the-scenes lobbying on behalf of Jewish refugees by Eleanor, Franklin Roosevelt's government issued protests but took little action beyond recalling its ambassador.

By 1939, when Roosevelt at last committed to taking on the isolationists of both parties, the hour was very, very late.

The Long Road to War: Japan

Japan's expansionism also had its roots in World War I, though in a somewhat different way. Japan had jumped into the European war only after the victors were clear, and had nonetheless reaped the benefits at the Versailles conference, which acknowledged Japan as a major regional power. Nationalists in Japan began to expound a vision of Japanese rule throughout Asia, following the European colonial model. They imbibed the pseudoscientific racism popular in Europe and America and adjusted it to make the Japanese the master race, destined to rule their genetically inferior neighbors. As in Germany, this belief in the sub-humanity of their victims would lead to massive atrocities by the Japanese army.

The pattern of political life in 1920s and '30s Japan was depressingly like that of Europe.

Moderate left-wing politicians were assassinated or frightened into leaving political life. The growing power of imperialists encouraged the formation of extreme left-wing groups, who in turn were cited by the imperialists as justification to assume more and more dictatorial powers. Emperor Hirohito's role in Japan's imperialism continues to be debated, but at a minimum it can be said that he did little to oppose its rise, and probably actively encouraged it.

In 1931, Japanese army officers launched a false-flag operation in the Chinese region of Manchuria, bombing a Japanese railway. The Japanese government then used this as a pretext to seize the entire province. President Hoover's Secretary of State, Henry Stimson, offered a rebuke but no action, encouraging later Japanese expansion.

Roosevelt made more efforts here than he would in the European crisis, but also to no avail. In 1934, he confidently asked the Senate to ratify a treaty admitted the United States to a World Court system, hoping that this would help rein in the Japanese. Isolationists including Huey Long and Father Coughlin went on the offensive, and Roosevelt was stunned to see the treaty scuttled. On July 7, 1937, continued tensions between Japan and China over the occupation of Manchuria flared into the Second Sino-Japanese War. (Some historians, particularly in Asian nations, consider this the proper start date of World War II, rather than the German invasion of Poland.) Japan took China's capital city, but Chinese Generalissimo Chiang Kai-Shek fell back and kept fighting; the armies fought back and forth until the 1945 Japanese surrender, claiming tens of millions of Chinese lives and millions of Japanese. Americans had long felt protective of China, the site of much Christian missionary activity, and Roosevelt was able to provide some aid to the Generalissimo. But direct military intervention was still out of the question.

Roosevelt vs. the Isolationists

As with earlier conservative/progressive splits, the foreign policy debates of 1930s America crossed party lines haphazardly and unpredictably. Because his own party contained both internationalists and isolationists, Roosevelt could follow neither path without splitting his coalition and risking the New Deal. When the Spanish Civil War broke out, for example, Roosevelt condemned fascist atrocities like the bombing of Guernica (immortalized in Pablo Picasso's painting of the same name), but made no move to aid the fascists' opponents. In 1937, he gave a speech calling for the world to "quarantine" aggressor nations without using military force--perhaps imagining what today we ~~would~~ call "sanctions"--but even on this he found little popular support.

Meanwhile, congressional isolationists had been working to bind the president's hands with a series of neutrality laws. A popular conspiracy theory of the time held that the U.S. had been manipulated into World War I by arms manufacturers; this theory was formally advanced by an investigatory committee headed by Senator Gerald Nye from 1934-36. Isolationists therefore not only passed laws forbidding the U.S. to join foreign conflicts, but even to sell munitions or provide material aid to nations at war, fearing that these actions would provoke enemy attacks. In 1938, with the international situation steadily worsening, Roosevelt sought modifications of these laws, but was defeated by Senate isolationists led by William Borah of Idaho. (Borah, as it happened, was a long-time lover of Franklin's cousin Alice Roosevelt--Eleanor's social nemesis (and Theodore's oldest daughter; he would later be famous for saying in late 1939, "Lord, if only I could have talked to Hitler, all this might have been averted.")

In September 1939, Germany invaded Poland, and even poor Neville Chamberlain--a decent, peace-loving man destined to be remembered as one of history's greatest suckers--realized that a world war could be postponed no longer. Britain and France declared war. Roosevelt reiterated American neutrality, but noted pointedly that "even a neutral cannot be asked to close his mind to conscience."

Roosevelt convened a special session of Congress and demanded the repeal of the arms embargo. For America to stay out of war, he argued, the nation must be prepared to help contain aggressor states. Failing to distinguish between aggressors and victims only meant that the aggressors could roll across the world unchecked, putting America in more jeopardy. Borah and the isolationists were reeling, having assured the public only weeks before that a full-scale European war was impossible, and public opinion swung solidly behind Roosevelt. Even the vigorous, deeply racist speeches of aviation hero Charles A. Lindbergh--one of the most respected Americans of his day--couldn't stop the president's momentum, and the arms embargo was modified to allow arms sales on a "cash and carry" basis.

With arms sales now permitted, Roosevelt began frantic efforts to move military supplies to Britain as quickly as possible. In May and June of 1940, Germany swept through Belgium, the Netherlands, Norway, Denmark, and France. The British army came to the brink of catastrophe at Dunkirk before being evacuated across the English Channel. Despite the heroic, bombastic rhetoric of new Prime Minister Winston Churchill, many in the American government and armed forces saw the British as a bad bet for American supplies, believing that war material was better invested in creating "Fortress America." Ambassador to Britain Joseph Kennedy (father to John F., Robert F., and Teddy) was blunt in his assessment that the British had no chance, as was Army Chief of Staff George Marshall. But Roosevelt ignored the advice of military planners, trusting in Churchill, and was vindicated by later events.

Roosevelt in '40

Suddenly Roosevelt no longer looked like the lame duck of the past two years. Under the traditional rules of American politics, though, he had little time left to act. George Washington had stepped down after two terms as president, despite his massive popularity, setting an important precedent for his successors in the belief that no one person should helm the nation for too long. A few presidents, including Ulysses S. Grant and Theodore Roosevelt, had seriously considered third terms since that time--Roosevelt actually pursuing one in 1912--but none had actually done so. Roosevelt had groomed Harry Hopkins as a potential successor throughout his second term, but Hopkins was now terminally ill. Vice President Garner, Postmaster General James Farley, and Secretary of State Cordell Hull all believed that they would be natural successors to FDR.

But with the world plunging into chaos, Roosevelt was reluctant to hand the reins of government to another--particularly a conservative like Garner or a man as uneducated about foreign affairs as Farley. Though he discussed his decision with no one, it gradually became clear that he would seek a third term for himself.

Meanwhile, the European war had thrown the Republicans into disarray. Their most obvious leaders, such as Ohio Senator Robert Taft or crusading New York attorney Thomas E. Dewey, were committed isolationists whose worldview looked increasingly foolish, even dangerous, to the general public. The Republicans finally made the unlikely choice of a conservative former Democrat from Indiana, Wendell Wilkie, who had changed his party allegiance only the year before. Wilkie's internationalist beliefs were so strong that he publicly offered Roosevelt support both in creating a draft and in sending destroyers to Great Britain, actions that would have been unthinkable just a few months before.

Roosevelt feigned indifference to a third term, but was soon "drafted" by the 1940 Democratic

National Convention, defeating Garner, Farley, and Hull on the first ballot by more than ten-to-one. He replaced Garner on the ticket with Secretary of Agriculture Henry A. Wallace, the far-left Iowa agrarian, hoping to lock up the farm belt and seeing him as a successor who would preserve the New Deal. (Given Wallace's embarrassing later apologetics for Stalin, well after a reasonable person should have had any doubts about the dictator's intentions, it's probably fortunate for the world that Roosevelt lived just long enough to replace Wallace on the ticket with Truman.) Roosevelt also undercut Wilkie's support by co-opting two internationalist elder statesmen of the Republican party, Henry Stimson and Frank Knox, into his cabinet. Stimson in particular would prove invaluable in the war effort to come, both as a master administrator and as a builder of bipartisan consensus.

Wilkie did better than Hoover or Landon before him, but still only carried ten states. Though public polls suggested Wilkie might have carried the country in a peacetime election, the voters overwhelmingly favored the experienced Roosevelt as their war president. Roosevelt would be returning for a full third term, the only American president ever to do so.

Lend-Lease

At the start of Roosevelt's third term, cash-and-carry was running into an unfortunate problem: the British were running out of cash. Roosevelt postponed the inevitable by making a destroyers-for-bases deal with Churchill, trading fifty destroyers for ninety-year leases to occupy British bases in the Caribbean and Canada. On December 29, 1940, Roosevelt announced his intention to have the United States become the "arsenal of democracy," equipping the Allies without American troops entering direct combat. But how to get the arsenal to the combatants?

The answer came to him on a Caribbean vacation that winter, and when he returned, he proposed Lend-Lease to the American public, a plan under which munitions would be "loaned" to Allied countries rather than sold. His metaphor became a famous example of his gift to translate geopolitics into everyday terms:

Let me give you an illustration: Suppose my neighbor's home catches fire, and I have a length of garden hose four or five hundred feet away. If he can take my garden hose and connect it up with his hydrant, I may help him to put out his fire. Now, what do I do? I don't say to him before that operation, "Neighbor, my garden hose cost me $15; you have to pay me $15 for it." What is the transaction that goes on? I don't want $15--I want my garden hose back after the fire is over.

Churchill joined the charade, declaring, "Give us the tools, and we will finish the job." The Lend-Lease program would continue throughout the war, and by the time the "fire" was out, Britain had received $31 billion in aid. Very little of this equipment ever found its way back to the U.S., of course--bullets, tanks and aircraft proved less re-usable than hoses--but it was a savvy end run around congressional restrictions.

Neither isolationists or internationalists had any illusions about where this was leading, however. Shipments of munitions to Britain would be fair game for German U-Boat attacks, and if the Germans began to sink American ships, American entry into the war was inevitable. This was a familiar scenario and indeed had been a prime cause of

America's entry into World War I. In the summer of 1941, Hitler unexpectedly opened a second front in his war, breaking his pact with Stalin in a surprise invasion of Russia. Despite some public grumbling in both countries, both Churchill and Roosevelt offered to make common cause with the hated Soviets, and the USSR was added to the Lend-Lease program.

By this point, Churchill's government had survived the aerial Battle of Britain, and the threat of German invasion was at least postponed if not over. But the threats of British starvation and shortages were very real; the nation simply could not provide for itself in the face of German attack. Thus began the Battle of the Atlantic, a desperate war of attrition in which Germany sought to sink merchant shipping faster than the Allies could sink U-boats. Still wary of provoking the isolationists, Roosevelt refused American captains permission to fire the first shot against German vessels, and even refused to declare war after American naval vessels were attacked and sunk. Despite an initial poor showing, the Battle of the Atlantic would eventually be won by the Allies, who transported enough supplies to keep Britain's war effort alive, but only at the cost of 3500 merchant vessels and 175 warships.

Meanwhile, in August 1941, Roosevelt and Churchill met to draft the Atlantic Charter, which began to plan for the postwar world. The document called for self-determination by all peoples, for global cooperation, and for a restoration of pre-war territorial boundaries. In this agreement lay the seeds of the future United Nations.

Infamy

Even as the conflict with Germany simmered, Roosevelt continued to escalate his support to

China. Japan had allied with Germany and attacked British and French possessions across Asia. Most of these fell quickly, in part due to racially-charged European arrogance; believing the Japanese to be cowardly and feeble "Orientals," the British were astonished to find themselves overrun by the brilliant, disciplined, and brutal Japanese war machine. Singapore soon fell, as did French Indochina (today's Vietnam). Invading under the slogan "Asia for the Asians," the Japanese were welcomed by resistance movements in every country, though these movements soon discovered that they had only traded one set of racist imperialists for another.

But for all its success, Japan was reliant on American oil, having little domestic supply. When Roosevelt responded to Japanese aggression by cutting off oil sales, its planners had few options left. They could withdraw, giving up their gains, or they could fight through British Malaysia and the American-held Philippines to the oil supplies of the East Indies (Indonesia). The war cabinet of Prime Minister Hideki Tojo chose the latter, gambling that the U.S. could be knocked out of the war with a single blow. The target: Pearl Harbor, a Hawaii naval base that housed much of the U.S. Pacific fleet.

The attack was perhaps the ultimate case of tactical victory but strategic disaster. Contrary to later conspiracy theories about Roosevelt's foreknowledge, the element of surprise was total--Roosevelt believed an attack was possible, even likely, but he expected it to come in the Philippines. The Japanese badly damaged all eight American battleships at Pearl Harbor, sinking four, as well as many smaller vessels, at the cost of only 64 Japanese casualties. The fighting was so one-sided that one never speaks of the "Battle of Pearl Harbor," only of the attack.

But Japan's triumph was illusory. In the possibly apocryphal words of Admiral Isoroku Yamamoto, Japan had only "awakened a sleeping giant," starting a war with a nation whose industrial capacity it could not hope to match. The attack, which Roosevelt famously called "the date which shall live in infamy," utterly failed in its objective of breaking the American resolve. Rather, the isolationist movement evaporated overnight. When Germany also declared war on the United States shortly after, Roosevelt at last had the public firmly behind him. He asked for, and received, formal declarations of war against both enemy nations. At last, the U.S. would fully join the war; the only question was if it had done so too late.

Choices at Home and Abroad

Though appalled at the losses, Churchill later recalled a feeling of intense relief after the

Pearl Harbor attack: "So we had won after all... There was no more doubt about the end... I went to bed and slept the sleep of the saved and thankful." Churchill

But the following months only saw further setbacks. The Japanese overran Douglas MacArthur's poorly prepared forces in the Philippines. Amazingly, and much to Roosevelt's fury, the general had failed to mobilize his defenses even after learning of the Pearl Harbor attack. But Roosevelt put political considerations ahead of justice in this instance and awarded MacArthur the Medal of Honor following a "daring escape" in which he abandoned his army to save himself and his general staff.

In the face of this continuing Japanese aggression, Roosevelt faced difficult choices about how to allocate America's resources. The Japanese were the more immediate threat, and were the only Axis nation to have attacked American soil. But Russia was buckling under the German invasion, and Stalin all but begged for the Allies to open a second front against Hitler. Churchill, too, saw Hitler as the greater threat; none of the Allies doubted that with Germany out of the war, Japan would quickly be defeated. After some consideration, Roosevelt agreed to this "Europe First" strategy.

Meanwhile, Roosevelt's War Department addressed the thorny issue of Japanese American citizens. A government report on Pearl Harbor set off national hysteria when it alleged without evidence that Japanese American spies and saboteurs had aided the attack, and the public clamored for action against this supposed enemy within. Roosevelt dodged the decision, delegating it Secretary of War Henry Stimson, who in turn passed the buck to James McCloy, a man who would become a postwar Establishment fixture. McCloy ordered more than 100,000 Japanese Americans rounded up into detainment camps, and--over Eleanor's public objections--Franklin formalized the policy with Executive Order 9066. These unlucky citizens found themselves forced to sell their property overnight, for losses of as much as $400 million, before being deported to live under guard in the bleak, makeshift camps. Roosevelt's executive order--later supported by a unanimous Congressional vote and two Supreme Court decisions--has been described as the greatest single civil rights violation in the history of the United States.

Fear of "Fifth Columnists" contributed to another tragedy as well. Refugees, particularly Jews, poured out of Europe in an endless stream. Just as today's politicians worry that ISIS will plant terrorists among the refugees fleeing their genocide, and therefore seek to close U.S. borders, Roosevelt and his war planners worried that the hordes of Jewish refugees from Nazi persecution might contain German spies or saboteurs. This fear battled with the president's humanitarian instincts, and he made only small-scale efforts to modify American immigration law. Tens of thousands of Jewish refugees were admitted by his efforts, but countless more were turned away, many of whom were repatriated and eventually killed in the German death camps. Roosevelt and Churchill have also been criticized for their failure to attack German death camps like Auschwitz later in the war, but this critique has much less justice. Even after they learned of the camps' existence, the Allied nations had few options to help. With the inaccurate bombing of the day, B-52s would have been lucky to drop a bomb within a half-mile of Auschwitz, much less specifically target the railroad lines or crematoria of the camps. Roosevelt and

Churchill were horrified by the scale of the Nazis' slaughter, but they believed the only way to stop it was to bring down the Third Reich itself.

Operation Torch

While Stalin angrily demanded that his allies to make an immediate, all-out assault on continental Europe to relieve pressure on Russia, Churchill--possibly concerned with maintaining Britain's colonial possessions--supported a policy of gradual encirclement, beginning by driving the Germans and Italians out of North Africa. General Marshall and other military planners bitterly opposed Churchill's plan on the grounds that North Africa had no strategic importance. But when they informed the president that a cross-Channel attack was still at least a year away, Roosevelt ordered them to go forward with a North African invasion, arguing that "U.S.

ground troops [must] be brought into action in 1942" to satisfy their allies and maintain the political momentum behind the war. (Reflecting years later, Marshall himself would retrospectively agree with the president's analysis.) The invasion was code-named Operation Torch and placed under the overall command of General Dwight D. Eisenhower.

As Rick Atkinson masterfully chronicles in An Army at Dawn, Roosevelt's decision also proved to be wise given the inexperience of American troops and officers, which led to debacle after debacle in the early phases of the North African fighting. Had these troops faced battle for the first time in an all-or-nothing attempt to secure a European beachhead, the consequences could have been much greater than they were. As it was, after months of hard fighting, the Allied forces defeated and secured the support of the local Vichy France government, drove the German forces of

General Erwin Rommel back into Tunisia, and encircled and destroyed them. By the time the American, British, and Free French forces pressed onto Italy, the Americans were a sturdier, experienced combat force led by able officers, the most notable of whom were the flamboyant cavalry officer George S. Patton and the "GI's general," Omar Bradley.

The subsequent Italian campaign would prove less of a success. Roosevelt was now splitting America's resources between a build-up for D-Day and the invasion of Italy, and both suffered as a result. Mussolini's government fell in the initial push, but the Germans proved harder to dislodge from Italy's mountainous terrain. Eager for results, Churchill talked Roosevelt into amphibious landings behind enemy lines at Salerno and Anzio, both of which were near-disasters that pinned down Allied forces for months. Italy claimed almost 200,000 American casualties, a fifth of the country's losses in the entire war, while making little progress in the ultimate fight against Germany.

Another less successful Roosevelt strategy was his heavy reliance on air power. For a president who had long been ambivalent about sending American ground troops into combat, aerial assault seemed like a logical alternative. Long before the Channel could be crossed, Americans could strike at German fortifications and manufacturing with long-range bombers. But strategic bombing turned out to be less successful and far more dangerous than Roosevelt's hopes early in the war, when he and some of his advisors believed that air power could win the war almost alone. Night-time raids made it almost impossible to reliably hit targets; day-time raids were took a brutal toll on the air crews. In 1943, two-thirds of all American airmen were killed or wounded before their tours of duty were complete. Accidents killed almost as many as did enemy fire. The massive bombing raids did slow German industrial production and transport, and historians remain divided as to their effectiveness. But the objective of diminishing enemy morale through bombing remained elusive. Just as the American had rallied rather than surrendering after Pearl Harbor, so too did the bombings of Tokyo and Berlin only increase the resolve of the populace. Had the Allies diverted these men and material into ground forces and tanks, it seems likely the war could have been brought to an earlier end.

War in the Pacific

The war against Japan began to turn in March 1942, when the Allies defeated an attempted invasion of Port Moresby, the capital of Papua New Guinea. For the remaining three years of the war, the Japanese would be in steady retreat. The crucial blow came in June, when the Japanese Navy was devastated in the Battle of Midway by an American fleet under the command of Admiral Chester Nimitz.

But despite the growing naval and aerial superiority of the Allies, the fight ahead was long and grueling. Both sides poured forces into the island of Guadalcanal in 1942 and '43, a battle eventually won by the Allies at great cost. MacArthur pursued a strategy of island-hopping toward the Japanese homeland, annihilating the Japanese strongholds one at a time. This strategy remains controversial among later analysts; MacArthur's approach was thorough, but also spent American lives to invade islands of little strategic significance. The remnants of the Japanese Navy were finished off in the Battle of the Philippine Sea and the Battle of Leyte Gulf, and with the Philippines reconquered, the US bombers began regular attacks against the Japanese mainland, including firebombings that devastated whole cities of paper-and-wood buildings.

The Home Front

Though the American people remained largely unified in the face of the foreign threat, Roosevelt still faced various challenges to his authority at home. In 1943, the nation's coal miners, led by John L. Lewis of the United Mine Workers, went on strike. When negotiations between the president and Lewis broke down, Roosevelt finally seized the mines under emergency war powers, and the miners went back to work. Despite this experience, however, Roosevelt vetoed the Smith-Connally Act that would have rolled back many New Deal gains for collective bargaining. (Congress nonetheless passed it over his veto.)

An even more serious threat came from the racial issues that Roosevelt had tried to suppress for so long. The dislocations of the war were bringing new groups into the American workforce. Most famous were the women who took jobs in industrial plants, forever symbolized by "Rosie the Riveter." But African Americans also found new jobs open to them, jobs once held only by whites. Trouble was inevitable. The worst of the subsequent riots was in Detroit, where in June 1943, tensions exploded into violence that killed 34, wounded more than a thousand, and did more than $2 million in property damage.

Meanwhile, black leaders were bringing increasing pressure to bear on Roosevelt for the way that some defense contractors excluded blacks from higher-paid positions. A. Philip Randolph of the Brotherhood of Sleeping Car Porters led the charge, threatening a 100,000-person protest march on Washington. Desperate to avert this, Roosevelt called Randolph and Walter White of the NAACP to the White House. When the pair proved implacable in their demands, Roosevelt signed Executive Order 8802, forbidding federal contractors to discriminate by race. It was the first step forward for civil rights in his presidency, or indeed in any presidency since Reconstruction. In return, Randolph and White agreed to call off their march.

D-Day

After the high costs and low returns of the Italian invasion, Roosevelt was at last finished with Churchill's "encirclement" strategy. The Americans were now providing the overwhelming majority of war material and an increasing amount of manpower, and Churchill could no longer treat Roosevelt as a junior or even equal partner. American plans called for the largest-ever amphibious landing in Normandy, and then a quick thrust for Germany's jugular. Despite some last-minute drama with the weather, the operation was carried out successfully in June 1944. The Allies were in back on the mainland of Europe, and rapidly rolled across France. In Italy, Rome finally fell. On the Eastern Front, Russians had broken the back of the German offensive at Kursk--the largest tank battle in the history of the world--and were also grinding toward Berlin.

It seemed possible that the war would be over by Christmas, and Eisenhower and British General Bernard Montgomery launched Operation Market Garden, a complex and daring operation to parachute behind enemy lines, seize a series of bridges, and pour into Germany in a single stroke. The Germans defeated the plan for now, but still the end was in sight. A shocking last German attempt to break the Allied line--later called the Battle of the Bulge--was defeated, and no one doubted that Hitler's end was at hand.

Postwar Planning

With the end of the war a foregone conclusion for at least two years before its formal end, Roosevelt devoted much of his time to shaping the world to come. In the Atlantic Charter, Roosevelt had been steadfast for the principle of self-determination, over which he and Churchill regularly clashed. Churchill at the time was ordering the imprisonment of Mahatma Gandhi and other leaders of the Indian independence movement, and he realized that Roosevelt's policy effectively meant the end of colonialism.

Churchill was also surprised and irked by Roosevelt's declaration at a January 1943 press conference that the Allies would accept nothing less than "unconditional surrender" from the Axis governments. Roosevelt's declaration was dramatic, but also dangerous. By shutting the door on a negotiated peace, it guaranteed a long war, particularly in the case of the Japanese, who believed the Americans would depose the emperor they worshipped as a god. Had the Allies rescinded this demand and accepted Japanese offers of conditional surrender, the atomic bombs need never have been used--an especially sad consideration when one remembers that MacArthur later decided to keep Hirohito on his throne regardless.

Roosevelt's most lasting contribution would be the creation of the United Nations. He had seen his hero Woodrow Wilson's League of Nations shattered by American isolationism and geopolitical pressures, and was determined to create an organization that could avoid the same mistakes. In 1942, the

Allied nations pledged to form a United Nations after the war, and began to refer to themselves by this title. More detailed plans were laid in a conference at Dunbarton Oaks in later 1944 under the leadership of Secretary of State Cordell Hull.

In meeting with his "Big Three" counterparts, Roosevelt appeared to be more trusting of Stalin than Churchill was, for which he has been widely criticized by later historians. When Churchill warned of the likelihood that Stalin would seize Eastern Europe, for example, Roosevelt replied that "I just have a hunch that Stalin is not that kind of a man." Shortly before his death Roosevelt came to see Stalin as the same bloody dictator that Churchill did, but it made little difference. Whether Roosevelt trusted Stalin or not, he had no realistic options available. Stalin would not have abandoned Poland and the rest of Eastern Europe without yet another war, and after two years of propaganda painting Russia as a stalwart ally, the exhausted American people might well have impeached any president who proposed pushing on from Berlin to Moscow in 1945. With the atomic bomb still untested, Roosevelt also believed he would need Stalin's help for a joint invasion of the Japanese mainland, which American planners believed could result in as many as a million casualties. Just as in 1943, to speak the truth about Stalin's tyranny would be to lose a needed ally. Roosevelt held his tongue.

Roosevelt in '44

In 1944, Roosevelt knew his re-election was virtually assured. The war was nearing victory, and the Republicans continued to be in disarray. He began to dream of another realignment of American politics, one in which he joined with his former challenger, Democratic apostate Wendell Wilkie, to create a new progressive party that had no need of conservative Southern Democrats for support. But news of the plan leaked prematurely, and Wilkie passed away unexpectedly of heart failure.

At the convention, party bosses forced Roosevelt drop the radical Wallace, and after some deliberation, Roosevelt settled on Harry S. Truman of Missouri as a running mate. Truman was a product of a Kansas City political machine, but had remained surprisingly clean himself, and had made a name for himself with his Senate committee to investigate waste in wartime planning. Despite Roosevelt's manifestly declining health, he and the party leaders put little thought into the selection or possible succession. Truman would never know much more about Roosevelt's plans for war and diplomacy than what he could read in the newspapers.

Against Roosevelt and Truman, the Republicans put up Thomas E. Dewey of New York, the prosecutor who had brought down the mobster Lucky Luciano. No one expected Dewey to have a real chance--it was more an audition for 1948, a year in which he would famously fight Truman down to the wire. After a campaign in which he ran on his record of war leadership and his support of the United Nations, Roosevelt won with 432 out of 531 electoral votes.

Last Visit to Warm Springs

In April 1944, Roosevelt took a badly needed vacation to his resort in Warm Springs, Georgia. Unknown to Eleanor, Franklin had invited Lucy Mercer Rutherfurd, the woman who had once broken up their marriage, to join him.

At one o'clock in the afternoon of April 12, Roosevelt was speaking with a butler when he jerked and said, "I have a terrific pain in the back of head." They would be his last words. He collapsed on the spot, and his doctors put him to bed. A chain smoker under tremendous stress, Roosevelt had experienced a massive stroke. Two hours later, he was dead.

Epilogue

Lucy Mercer Rutherfurd was whisked away from the scene of Roosevelt's death, and her presence did not become public knowledge until 1966, when an FDR aide named Jonathan W. Daniels published a memoir. But Eleanor learned within weeks of her old rival's presence; without meaning to, Franklin had hurt Eleanor one last time after all.

Meanwhile, the Allied nations mourned. Church bells rang, and soldiers wept. Winston Churchill was devastated by Roosevelt's death, believing his friend had done more than any other man to save the free world from fascism and was "the greatest man I've ever known." Even Stalin was reportedly moved by the news. Meanwhile, Harry Truman assumed the presidency, coming to the job so ill-informed that he had never even heard of the atomic bomb he would soon have to decide whether or not to drop. Despite all political predictions, he was a somewhat successful president, and eked out a close win against Dewey in 1948 to be elected to the presidency in his own right. His second term allowed another four years for Roosevelt's New Deal to cement into political permanence.

Eleanor Roosevelt carried on in politics. She served for years as the American delegate to the UN General Assembly and played a key role in drafting that body's Universal Declaration of Human Rights. She fought on for civil rights, at times traveling through the South with a loaded gun in case of trouble; the FBI had warned her that the Ku Klux Klan had actively called for her assassination. When she died in 1962, she was popularly remembered not as First Lady of the nation, but as "First Lady to the World."

Franklin Delano Roosevelt's complicated legacy continues to shape, and occasionally to haunt, America. The debate over the Roosevelt

Memorial itself was typical. Planners wanted a statue of Roosevelt standing--Roosevelt as he wished the public to see him--while disabled groups wanted a statue of Roosevelt in his wheelchair: Roosevelt as he actually was. Neither side conclusively won that fight. Neither side ever will.

Sources

Atkinson, Rick. An Army at Dawn. New York: Henry Holt, 2002.

Brands, H.W. Traitor to His Class: The Privileged Life and Radical Presidency of Franklin Delano Roosevelt. New York: Doubleday, 2008.

Cook, Blanche Wiesen. Eleanor Roosevelt: 1884-1933. New York: Penguin, 1992.

Daniels, Roger. Franklin D. Roosevelt: Road to the New Deal, 1882-1939. Chicago: U of Illinois Press, 2015.

Franklin D. Roosevelt Presidential Library and Museum.http://www.fdrlibrary.marist.edu/. Accessed March 2016.

Goodwin, Doris Kearns. No Ordinary Time: Franklin and Eleanor Roosevelt: The Home

Front in World War II. New York: Simon & Schuster, 1994.

Johnson, Paul. A History of the American People. London: Weidenfeld & Nicholson, 1997.

Kennedy, David M. Freedom From Fear: The American People in Depression and War, 1929-45. New York: Oxford UP, 1999.

Manchester, William. The Glory and the Dream: A Narrative History of America, 1932-72. Boston: Little, Brown, and Co., 1973.

Miller, Nathan. F.D.R.: An Intimate History. New York: Doubleday, 1983.

Oshinsky, David M. Polio: An American Story. New York: Oxford UP, 2005.
Smith, Jean Edward. FDR. New York: Random House, 2007.

Tobin, James. The Man He Became: How FDR Defied Polio to Win the Presidency. New York: Simon & Schuster, 2013.

Made in the USA
Monee, IL
18 August 2020